R07966

DATE DUE

MAR 2 1982	JUN 0 2 2008
FEB 27 1991	
JUL 1 1 1994	
OCT 1 6 1994	
DEC 4 1995	

5'82   S-180

HCP-301   F94
HCP-301   F96

The End
of Medicine

HEALTH, MEDICINE, AND SOCIETY:
A WILEY-INTERSCIENCE SERIES
DAVID MECHANIC, Editor

The End
of Medicine

RICK J. CARLSON

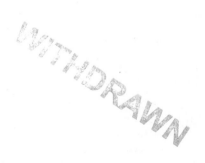

A WILEY-INTERSCIENCE PUBLICATION

JOHN WILEY & SONS

New York · London · Sidney · Toronto

Library of Congress Cataloging in Publication Data

Carlson, Rick J
    The end of medicine.

    (Health, medicine, and society)
    "A Wiley-Interscience publication."
    Bibliography: p.
    Includes index.
    1. Medical care—United States. 2. Medical innovations. 3. Social medicine. 4. Hygiene. I. Title.
[DNLM: 1. History of medicine. 2. Philosophy, Medical. W61 C284e]

RA395.A3C36   362.1′0973   75-6856
ISBN 0-471-13494-5

Printed in the United States of America

10 9 8 7 6 5

Foreword

By training, Carlson is a lawyer. He has chosen to prosecute medicine. Unlike other members of the legal profession who have recently taken up class actions in which medical institutions are indicted, Carlson argues in defense of society as a whole and urges nothing less than the dissolution of the contemporary health care system. There is no precedent for a jeopardy of this magnitude. Carlson urges the disestablishment rather than the reorganization or expropriation of the largest social service system the world has known. The thrust of his argument is both politically and technically so radical that it does not fit any of the major constellations into which the criticism of medicine had crystallized by the early seventies, both in America and in Western Europe.

Carlson argues that the system of engineering interventions on people and on environments, which constitutes the contemporary medical endeavor and around which the modern medical institution is built, has almost no relevance to health. He marshals a host of firsthand witnesses for evidence on this point. He shows that the widespread presumption of benefits derived by society from increasing medical expenditures is based on misguided trust in scientific hearsay given by professionally prejudiced testimony.

But Carlson goes further. He argues convincingly that the very limited net benefits to public health that the health profession now can still credibly claim must disappear during the next 25 years, while social costs and damages generated by the medical complex will become literally sickening. Nobody so far has shown with comparable cogency that this inevitably growing counterproductivity of the United States health care system is fundamentally independent of any changes in medical education, technological progress, and organizational streamlining or any of the political alternatives to the control of health care now under discussion.

Over several decades the United States public has progressively granted an almost total autonomy to its medical establishment, which came to govern an increasing proportion of the total population, by defining sickness, by recognizing the sick, and by deciding what shall be done to them. Now that that autonomy has turned into a unique kind of monopoly and now that patient relationships in the United States outnumber the population, a political consensus is emerging that the Legislature shall formally contract this hygienic hierarchy for the therapeutic tutelage of the people.

Carlson provides support for the minority position which, based on the spirit of the First Amendment, challenges the uninformed consensus which makes the establishment of a medical church highly probable.

Carlson wants to be heard before the almost inevitable legal enactment of this new establishment freezes the style of present health care and with it our spent civilization. He knows that he cannot be heard if he sticks to the prosecution of medicine and to the discrediting of its merely technical or political reformists. He believes that to get a hearing on his substantive argument he should risk references to alternative forms of health care. He does so to give some concrete content to the alternative policies that he proposes.

CIDOC   IVAN ILLICH
Cuernavaca, Mexico

Series Editor's Preface

The End of Medicine by Rick Carlson argues that a new paradigm is emerging in health services, and that its encouragement is essential. We do not anticipate that the reader will accept all his assumptions or all of the evidence that he provides in support of his view. As Carlson himself suggests, his view is personal, and some of his arguments are idiosyncratic, unconventional, and occasionally esoteric. His book in part represents an entry into unknown regions, where the evidence or possibilities remain vague. But we are confident that his discussion of the end of medicine will stimulate readers to consider and clarify their own assumptions, whether for the purpose of traveling Carlson's path, or seeking to disown it.

Much of the ferment in the health field arises from the somewhat different perspectives of those professionals who design, provide, and evaluate health services, and laypersons who increasingly demand greater voice in establishing priorities and assessing the performance of our social institutions. There are growing criticisms of professional dominance and expert opinion, which are alleged to have contributed to many of our current social crises and to have limited approaches to societal problems by their commitment to narrow and specialized technologies, rather than to a larger social and ecological perspective. Although it remains to be seen to what extent these criticisms of the expert are valid, or to what extent they reflect the discomfort of living in an increasingly complex and dynamic society, it is apparent that differences of viewpoint help us clarify our assumptions and practices. The layperson's perspective provides another view of health, which may open up possibilities that professionals have failed to see or have ignored.

The Wiley-Interscience series Health, Medicine, and Society is devoted to examining the relationships between health and other social institutions, the assumptions of medical practice, and the historical, sociocultural, and technological forces that affect the evolution of medicine and health care more generally. For the most part, books in this series are written by social and behavioral scientists, physicians, and analysts from the fields of public health and government. They all come to the health arena with assumptions and perspectives that have been shaped in part by their professional socialization and the current trends of thinking in their respective fields.

But we shall occasionally open the series to examinations by laypersons who have a special interest in medicine and health, and how the two are practiced. We do so with the understanding that they are not "scientific" discussions in the same sense as some of our more technical volumes, but that they raise issues and questions that deserve public discussion. We feel that it is important that professionals and laypersons communicate with one another about their assumptions and expectations of patients and health professionals, that they make some effort to grasp one another's perspectives, and that they educate one another when they find no sound basis for the other's views. We hope that the opportunity for such a dialogue in this series will stimulate new areas of inquiry and research that provide a more sound basis for the organization and provision of health services in the future.

A word about Rick Carlson himself. Mr. Carlson is an attorney, who following his training became involved in the development of health legislation. He played a role in the formulation and examination of the concept of the Health Maintenance Organization as a staff member of the Institute for Interdisciplinary Studies (now Inter-Study), a nonprofit research organization. As a lawyer with little background in health, who found himself in the midst of formulating health legislation, Rick Carlson began to ask questions, and read widely to develop a better understanding of the goals of health legislation and how they might best be promoted. This was the trigger that led him, while a Visiting Fellow at the Center for the Study of Democratic Institutions, to write this book as an answer to some of his own concerns. He was not satisfied with the role of technician, but sought to clarify for himself the goals toward which the total effort of the medical care system was being generated. It is particularly valuable for persons involved in the policy-formulation process to so openly expose themselves, to express their thoughts, questions, and assumptions. For it is only through the self-corrective process of dialogue and understanding that the policy-maker who formulates and administers legislation, the health professional who provides the service, and the client, who is the object of it all, can develop a better appreciation of one another's role and perspectives.

DAVID MECHANIC
Center for Advanced Study
in the Behavioral Sciences,
Stanford, California

Preface

This book is personal. I am not a health scientist, as many may delight in telling me when they have read what I have to say. Yet I am not unacquainted with the subject of medical care. As a health services researcher for more than three years, I examined the means by which medical care is provided. Consequently, I became acquainted with many physicians and other health scientists and with medical care issues. My admiration for the complexity of the subject grew, as did my admiration for many of the professionals laboring to make the system better. But one question persisted, one that everyone seemed to ignore: what impact did medical care have on health? But there was no time to pursue the issue.

In late 1972 and during most of 1973 I was a Visiting Fellow at the Center for the Study of Democratic Institutions, Santa Barbara. Although other projects intruded, I finally found the time to examine the question and found an answer that surprised me: medical care had very little to do with health. But since the evidence, although convincing, was sparse, I took up three other questions. First, if medical care has little to do with health, what does have to do with it? Second, if the relationship between medicine and health is tenuous, why have we created such a large and costly system to provide medical care? And finally, is there something faulty about the way we think about health?

These questions launched my work. This book deals with them in the order in which they are raised here.

This book is also personal because some of the arguments, particularly in the last few chapters, are idiosyncratic. Some of the material is unconventional, and occasionally esoteric. But it characterizes my view of the world and bares my value preferences. The way that I view the world necessarily influences my perception of medicine's place in it. These latter arguments may be less tenable to some readers than those offered in other parts of the book. And although they are important, and to some indispensable, other readers may decide that the argument is complete without them. To me, however, they are integral. For in my view, real change, in medicine and health as in anything else, cannot be accomplished without a radical transformation of humanity.

RICK J. CARLSON

Santa Barbara, California
Aspen, Colorado
December 1974

Contents

1

Introduction

The end of medicine is near. Medical care as provided by physicians and hospitals is having less and less impact on our health. This will become more clear in the next few decades, perhaps by the year 2000.

Our contemporary approach to medical care in the United States is only one road that has been traveled in the history of health care—and possibly a blind alley. There are, in general, five ways to approach the generation of health. The first approach assumes that the health of both populations and individuals is beyond the control of mortals, and thus subject to the whims of the supernatural. The second, in which the emphasis is on the health of populations, can be roughly characterized as a "public health" approach. This approach stresses interventions into the social and environmental orders; its intent is to foster conditions that prevent disease and are conducive to health. Related to the second approach is a third, which also emphasizes "prevention" but is distinguishable in that it focuses on individual patients rather than populations. The fourth, or "natural" approach to health, embraces the second and third but stresses the self-limiting nature of disease and the role of the individual in achieving health. Fifth and finally, health can be sought principally through services that are delivered by a medical care system designed to treat the "symptoms" of illness.

Medicine in the Western world, and particularly in the

United States where it is the most elaborate, falls into the last category. In other words, in modern medical practice the doctor awaits the appearance of illness in a patient and then intervenes through the use of profound tools such as surgery and chemotherapy. But although modern medicine can cure and by so doing can restore health, the limits of medicine have been reached.

THE ARGUMENTS

My first thesis is that the impact of medical care on health is substantially less than the public assumes. The second thesis follows from the first. When placed in a social, economic, and environmental context, our medical care system has less impact on health than social and environmental factors have, and will have even less impact in the future. A case against medical care can be made knowing what we know today, but an examination of selected trends in society—a set of possible "social futures"—reveals a widening divergence between what medical care can do and the needs of the public 25 years from now.

These theses lead to a third: We must start over in our efforts to achieve health. This will require new thinking and new approaches, and it will also require abandoning much of the system that now provides medical care. We should preserve those elements of the existing service system that work. But we must also be revolutionary because the resources that will be needed to try new approaches are currently harnessed to a sophisticated, professionalized medical care system which, in the interests of aiding the few, sacrifices the health of the many.

Within the next few years, Congress will enact a program of national health insurance. This legislation will underwrite the costs of care for all citizens of the United States. But if it can be shown, for example, that spending a dollar on education would improve health more than spending the same dollar on health services, or if it could be demonstrated that diet and nutrition are far more important to health than any amount of curative care, the need for a national health insurance program becomes doubtful.

Congress will not face these issues. But it should. The issues should be of vital interest to those interested in fiscal austerity and lean government, as well as to those who feel that health is of the greatest national importance, irrespective of cost. Should we indenture our health in the future to the existing medical care system when better health might be ensured through other means? The answer should be no; but it is virtually certain that Congress will do so, and with the support of the vast majority of the people.

The argument in this book, then, is profoundly radical, even revolutionary. It calls for the dissolution of the largest and most expensive social service system in the world—the medical care system in the United States. But my critique diverges from the usual radical critique of medical care. The "radical" critique centers first on the exploitation of the hapless consumer by the rapacious provider and, second, on the failure of the "system" to extend services to everyone, in spite of the alleged exploitation. This analysis is accurate as far as it goes, but it fails to engage the pivotal issue—what does medicine have to do with health? The radical solution—the provision of care to everyone—may simply result in more care for those who may not need it. But if it is health we care about, and not medical care, we must look for improvements in the life setting of the unhealthy, not simply the provision of services designed to cure them once they are sick.

People must relearn how to take care of themselves and one another. Further, they must learn how to use providers as resources. If this can be done, then a leaner and tougher approach to health can be created out of the remains of the current delivery system. The new approach will build on

those things that generate health; unlike present-day
medicine, it will not rely on profound interventions when
health has been lost.

The Order of the Arguments. The United States is about to
enter into a "contract" with the existing medical care delivery system by legislating its legitimacy through a national
health insurance program. This might be a fatal step. Consequently, the chapters to follow march to a strident beat. I
begin with evidence on the relative impact of personal medical care and a set of socioenvironmental factors. It is here, in
Chapter 2, that much of the research and literature on the
"effectiveness" of medical care is compiled. Then I turn to a
history of the "crisis" in health care, together with a discussion of its evolutionary features, to show where and how it is
evolving. Next I turn to some "social futures" for the United
States and their implications for health. This is done dialec-
tically, by contrasting the evolution of medicine with a projection of the future, to demonstrate the divergence between
the medical care system and the larger society of which it is a
part.

In Chapter 5, I synthesize my points to argue for the "end
of medicine." But this chapter also adds some new dimensions. The end of medicine is coming both because of internal contradictions within the present system and because the
system does not correspond with an emerging zeitgeist.

The final two chapters draw things together. In Chapter
6, I attempt to state what health is, having spent five chapters spelling out what it is not. In Chapter 7, through a brief
historical analysis of the eras of medicine, I propose some of
the elements of a new paradigm for health. In this last
chapter I also resurrect the question of national health insurance, because it is on this question that the public debate
about health care will turn. If a comprehensive program of
national health insurance is promulgated in the next few

years, as is almost certain, the structure, prerogatives, and style of practice of the existing medical care system will be frozen for decades. If the outcome is simply more medical care, our health will be worse and our well-being as a population will be in jeopardy.

Finally, in an epilogue I draw the broad outlines of a new medicine, which must be calibrated with the future and specifically with the health care needs of the future.

The arguments in this book are fundamentally theoretical in nature. Although most of the points are documented, the ultimate test is their theoretical strength. This book is only a prospectus for the hard empirical work that should be done.

2

The Impact
of Medicine

Voltaire suggested that "the efficient physician is the man who successfully amuses his patient while nature effects a cure."

Medicine is a conundrum to those who have not had medical training. Three characteristics of medical practice are particularly perplexing to the uninitiated.

First, determinations of the quality of care are made without reference to the actual outcomes of care to the patient. To use a homely example, most of us judge a restaurant on the basis of the taste and quality of the food. Seldom do we inquire as to the chef's lineage or education, or visit the kitchen to inspect the ovens and utensils. The quality of means and the results of health care are matters of different importance and magnitude, but the analogy fits. Unlike the quality of food, the regulatory measures traditionally employed to control the quality of medical care have focused on who renders it and how, more often than on what the results have been.

There is one notable exception, although Florence Nightingale should get similar kudos. In the early 1900s, Dr. E. A. Codman, a surgeon at Massachusetts General Hospital, sought to orient assessment of the quality of medical care from structural or input evaluation—who did it—to process

and end-result evaluation—how and why.[1] But first he had
to find out what was going on. He started by monitoring 692
hospitals of 100 or more beds. The results revealed shock-
ingly low quality of care; only 89 of the 692 hospitals could
meet the standards established for the study. Limited circulation of the results aroused so much controversy that Codman could not at first get his findings published and then
could not find sponsors for further research.

Codman's approach was radical and would still be viewed
that way today. He argued that patients should be required
to pay only for good results, and that people should be
aware of the results of their care. This is a slight variation on
the practice in Babylon of severing the physician's hand if he
failed to cure. Codman practiced his beliefs. He published
annual reports that documented the results of his care and
his methods of accounting for the results. For example, of
the 337 cases he treated between 1911 and 1917, Dr. Codman concluded that 183 (or 54 percent) were managed
without undue complications. For the remaining 154 cases
that were not satisfactorily managed in his judgment, 204
separate judgments were made to determine why problems
arose. In most cases (roughly 76 percent), the problems were
found to be due to errors in physician care, including surgical misjudgment, use of faulty equipment, or misdiagnosis.

Second, and more puzzling than the failure of the medical
care enterprise to examine its results, is the paucity of research on the impact of care on the health of populations.
Controlled clinical trials have been used to measure the
impact of medical cures for individual patients. But, historically, with the surrender of medicine to the scientific
method, "population" medicine was relegated to the schools
of public health, while medicine went to work on the individual. Consequently, we know something about medicine's
impact on individual patients but very little about the impact
of medical care on populations.

Third, there is even less research on the *relative* impact of personal medical care services and other socioenvironmental factors such as education, housing, air, water, seat belts, and Muzak. In other words, other than some anecdotal and impressionistic evidence, we have virtually no information on the relative weight to assign to the various factors that bear on health, including medical care. In part, this is due to the confusion of medical care with health.

This chapter takes up the impact question. First, evidence about the outcomes of medical care, when it is presumed to be efficacious, is examined. Then the obverse is examined—when the outcomes are adverse as a result of iatrogenesis, or disease "caused" by the medical care system itself. Next, the placebo effect is assessed, followed by a discussion of the importance of caring. The balance of the chapter examines the slender research on the impact of medical care on the health of populations and concludes with a review of the even more sparse work on the relative impact of medical care and other factors on health.

To grapple with this subject, the following definitions developed by the World Health Organization can be used. "Efficacy" is the benefit or utility to the individual of the service, treatment regimen, drug, or preventive or control measures advocated or applied. "Effectiveness" is the effect of the activity and the end results, outcome, or benefits for the population achieved in relation to the stated objectives. "Efficiency" is the efforts or end results achieved in relation to the effort expended in terms of money, resources, and time.

THE IMPACT OF MEDICAL CARE ON PATIENTS

The Outcomes of Medical Care. There is mounting evidence that the quality of medical care is uneven. There is also evidence that it is poor in a surprisingly high number of instances. But we lack a comprehensive body of research.

The Center for the Study of Responsive Law incorporated much of the research that has been done in its publication, *One Life—One Physician.*[2]

One illustration in the book is the work of Dr. Charles E. Lewis, then of the Harvard Center for Community Health and Medical Care, now at UCLA. Dr. Lewis reviewed the records of the Kansas Blue Cross Association over a one-year period (only two hospitals in the state failed to participate in the review). He tabulated the number of elective operations for removal of tonsils, hemorrhoids, and varicose veins, and the operations for hernia repair, in all the hospitals in each of the state's 11 regions. Variations for the average rate of these four elective surgical procedures ranged from a low of 75 operations per 10,000 persons in one region to a high of 240 operations per 10,000 persons in another. Striking variations were also found between regions within each elective surgical category. The high and low regional incidences (rounded off) per 10,000 persons were: for tonsillectomy, 153 and 432; for hemorrhoidectomy, 11 and 35; for varicose veins, 3 and 7; and for hernia repair, 18 and 43.[3]

Some of this variation can be explained by differences in patient income, disease incidence, number of physicians, and so forth. There is little doubt, however, that part of the variation is due to the relationship between the medical care provided and the number and type of providers providing it. This relationship can be illustrated by looking at rates of surgery. In the United States, there are twice as many surgeons in proportion to population as in England and Wales. And there is twice as much surgery in the United States as in England and Wales.[4]

Another major study, the National Halothane Study, after adjusting for age, sex, year, diagnosis, physical status, and previous operations, revealed threefold variations in postoperative mortality among 34 distinguished teaching hospitals.[5] Despite this variation in mortality—a very real matter—physicians generally refuse to tell patients about to undergo surgery what anesthesia will be used and what the hospital's track record is in patient recovery. If the results of the Halothane study are accurate, many patients are rolling dice with their lives when they seek care.

Other evidence included in *One Life—One Physician* is equally unsavory. In general, the research shows that the quality of medical care varies greatly; many instances of poor care can be found. The data are also remarkable in light of the presuppositions most consumers hold about the quality and reliability of medical care. There is a limitation, however. Most of the studies in the report judge the quality of care by examining the "processes" of care rather than "outcomes" of care. In other words, the "manner" in which care was provided is the focus of most of the studies, rather than the actual "outcomes" of care.

There are few studies on "outcomes." One of the few studies in this emerging area of investigation was conducted by Robert H. Brook, M.D., and Robert L. Stevenson.[6] The outcomes for 141 emergency room patients were examined. Initially, only 94 of the 141 patients completed the battery of studies based on diagnostic X-rays; 77 (or 55 percent) received an adequate work-up based on the intern's diagnostic impression; but only 37 of 98 patients, having received diagnostic X-ray examinations, were informed whether the findings were normal or abnormal; and only 14 of the 38 patients with abnormal X-ray results (or 37 percent) appeared to have received adequate therapy for the conditions indicated. Thus, the study resulted in effective medical care for only 38 patients (or 27 percent). Ineffective care was given to 84 patients (or 60 percent). Neither effective nor ineffective care was given to 19 patients, or the remaining 13 percent.

The study was not conducted in a small rural hospital, nor in the inadequate and shabby facilities often found in major public hospitals. It was conducted in the Baltimore City

Hospital emergency room, where it was assumed that the competence and efficiency of the house staff would be optimal.[7] In terms of staffing ratios, quality of patient care, and evaluation efforts, the assumption was that the Baltimore City Hospital emergency room was the equal of any facility in the city of Baltimore, and perhaps of any in the United States.

At the time of the study, Dr. Brook was a postdoctoral student at Johns Hopkins School of Medicine. Although few doubts were expressed by his superiors about his methodology, the uncritical assumption was that the findings of the study were characteristic of City Hospital, a less prestigious institution than Johns Hopkins. The challenge proved too much for Brook; his next target was the emergency room at Johns Hopkins. Using essentially the same methodology, Brook's work revealed that only 28 percent of 166 patients with gastrointestinal symptoms were given acceptable care, 2 percent less than in the City Hospital.[8] It is a credit to the gentility of Johns Hopkins (or perhaps its relief) that Dr. Brook was graduated shortly thereafter.

In another study, David Kessner, M.D., used "tracer" methods to follow the treatment of one disease condition through the treatment system. His results were not unlike Brook's. He found that treatment was very checkered. And, although he has refrained from generalizing about his results, that is, from drawing inferences about medical care in general from treatment of the "tracer" condition, generalization seems warranted.[9] John Williamson employed predictive techniques to assess the physician's skill at relating the processes used to the outcomes of care to the patient. The findings do not foster an image of the physician as seer.[10] Still other significant studies have been undertaken by Mildred Morehead, Barbara Starfield, Laurence Weed, and others.[11] The sobering conclusion is that medicine is not the well-honed instrument it is generally thought to be. Inevitable human error abounds, and this is understandable. Less

understandable is medicine's persistent refusal to examine
what it does for the patient in relation to the result to the
patient.

*Iatrogenesis: How Patients Get More Than They Bargained
For.* Every August more tonsils are removed than in any
other month of the year. There are a number of reasons
why this occurs, but a principal one is that the physicians
need to keep busy. Tonsillectomy is the most common surgical procedure performed in Western civilization.[12] The procedure is used for various conditions for which removal of
the tonsils appears to be the cure; unfortunately, tonsillectomy often seems to be a ritual. According to Dr. A. Frederick North, Jr., visiting professor of Pediatrics at the University of Pittsburgh, "Ninety to ninety-five percent [of the
procedures] are unnecessary."[13] In a recent study, existing
data on the performance of tonsillectomy were scrutinized.
No compelling evidence of any long-term benefits was
discovered.[14] Under the most favorable conditions, no more
than 2 to 3 percent of children require tonsillectomy.
Nevertheless, recent data reflect that, in most communities,
approximately 20 to 30 percent have their tonsils removed.[15]

A more important issue is what possible risks and dangers
are experienced by those who undergo surgery. The mortality rate is low, about 1:1000 patients. Nonetheless, because
of the volume of cases, tonsillectomies account for 100 to
300 deaths annually in the United States. Serious complications occur in 15.6:1000 cases per year. Finally, there is some
evidence that removal of the tonsils results in the loss to the
patient of an invaluable "immunity" mechanism, possibly
linked to increased risk of Hodgkin's disease and bulbar
poliomyelitis.[16]

But the most important complications may be emotional.
The young tonsillectomy candidate, perhaps five or six years
of age, is made captive in a hospital, separated from his or

her parents, and surrounded by mysterious figures in white coats. The emotional harm is demonstrable, and the palliative ice cream at the end of surgery hardly compensates. The psychiatric literature contains evidence that childhood tonsillectomy often has profound irreversible and lifelong repercussions.[17]

Children's tonsils are not the only targets. Normal ovaries are also often needlessly removed. There is an extensive literature on this subject, most of which has been ignored by practitioners. Two studies are illustrative. The subtitle of the first speaks for itself: "A Study Based on Removal of 704 Normal Ovaries from 546 Patients." (One wonders which of the women lost more than one normal ovary.) In the second study, the investigators established surgical justification based on postoperative or pathological examination in only 54.9 percent of 6960 cases.[18]

Still other patients suffer injuries through the administration of drugs or the use of procedures which have unanticipated side effects. Classic examples of calamities in medicine have been the loss or impaired hearing of some patients given chloramphenicol, and the wrenching results of the use of thalidomide.[19] Moreover, infections contracted in hospitals exceed the rate in the average household, despite elaborate safety and hygiene measures. They include postoperative pulmonary infections, wound infections, burn infections, and tracheotomy infections, to name a few.

Catastrophes occur outside the hospital as well. Some recently concluded research links the death of thousands of asthmatics to the inhalation of isoprotermol, a medication for the treatment of asthma, which can be purchased either with a prescription or over the counter. Dr. Paul Stolley of the School of Hygiene and Public Health at Johns Hopkins University, in reviewing research on the question, remarked, "It's the most tragic drug disaster on record. There's nothing else—even thalidomide—that ranks with it."[20] The physicians who prescribed the drug and the drug company that marketed it undoubtedly expected the drug to relieve a common ailment. But that is not what happened. In England, the deaths of approximately 3500 asthmatics have been traced to its use.

Adverse results from tonsillectomies and hysterectomies, and infections are the most common iatrogenic phenomena, but there are others. Seymour Handler, M.D., in his article, "Bring Back the Mustard Plaster," lists some others.[21] One of the worst dangers for the unsuspecting patient is chemotherapy. Handler includes a table in his article matching modern medicinals with diseases that drugs can introduce:

Drug	*Disease*
Enteric coated KCI	Small intestine stenotric ulcers
Methysergide	Retroperitoneal fibrosis
Warfarin	Intramural intestinal hemorrhage
Tetracycline	Pediatric tooth discoloration
Nitrofurantoin	Pulmonary infligrates
Long-acting sulfonamides	Stevens-Johnson syndrome
Hydralizine, procainamide	Lopus enythematosus

This list is remindful of Immanuel Kant's observation that "Physicians think they are doing something for you by labeling what you have as a disease." Other iatrogenic procedures and practices listed by Handler include polypharmacy, the overprescribing of drugs for some patients. Charlotte Muller, a professor of urban studies at City University of New York, has extensively studied drug prescribing and use patterns. She documents the staggering degree of overmedication, and concludes that it is "one source of reduced human welfare."[22] Handler adds that the diagnosis of "nondisease" or, in other words, the erroneous determination by the physician that a disease is present when it is not, often results in needless restrictions to patients. Damage arising both from faulty diagnostic and therapeutic procedures is another example. Handler also spotlights a new and fascinating problem, psychosemantics, a congeries of anxieties induced in patients by what a physician says or implies.[23]

John Pekkanen examined the links between the pharmaceutical industry and medicine in his book, *The American Connection*.[24] Pekkanen examines drug advertisements addressed to physicians in widely read and respected journals such as the *New England Journal of Medicine* and the *Journal of the American Medical Association*. Amphetamines, tranquilizers like Valium and Librium, are the big sellers. New drugs are introduced to the market with an advertising barrage focused on the physician. Doctors are literally inundated by pharmaceuticals and pharmaceutical ads. Their journals, even the more popular ones like *Medical Economics* and *Medical World News*, are filled with them. Doctors' offices and probably their homes are well stocked with drugs, many proffered free by pharmaceutical companies. And then there are the grinning drug pushers—the detailers of the major pharmaceuticals. Since doctors do not have the time to educate themselves about most drugs, they frequently look to the detailer for their information. Pekkanen puts it this way:

> Contrary to their accepted image and contrary to what the public rightly expects, doctors often know very little about the drugs they are prescribing. Too often all they know is precisely what the drug companies want them to know. . . . He relies on the detail men, those ambassadors of good will from the industry. . . .[25]

There are unquestionably effective drugs, effectively prescribed. But there are also drugs like isoproternal and thalidomide that kill and maim. There are drugs that dull, like tranquilizers, and others that speed up, like the friendly amphetamine family. Doctors who seek to calm the frenzied

patient with tranquilizers and to bolster the will of the over-
weight patient with amphetamines are not necessarily harm-
ing the patients. But physicians who maintain a patient on
drugs because they are unwilling to consider alternatives
may be.

Iatrogenesis is a larger problem than malpractice. There is
ample evidence of malpractice—that is, error due to simple
negligence. A study completed in 1973 shows that, conservatively, 7 percent of all patients suffer compensable injuries
while hospitalized, but few of these patients do anything
about it.[26] The word "iatrogenesis" was coined to refer to
damage caused by the medical care system itself, often unanticipated, but including more than that arising out of the
negligence of practitioners. Infections, overmedication,
removal of healthy organs are all included, but a more
penetrating example is the diagnosis and treatment of "non-
disease."

Among the more common errors made in medicine is
diagnostic error. The assumption is that the error arises
from a false diagnosis, or from a failure to diagnose. But
error also arises when a problem is diagnosed that does not
exist. Heart murmurs can be "detected" in up to one-half of
a given sample of children. For example, in one investigation, 44.4 percent of 4039 Nashville schoolchildren had "in-
nocent" murmurs.[27] Unfortunately, heart "murmur" is often
confused with heart "disease." In a study of 20,800 Seattle
schoolchildren, 93 were identified as having heart disease or
rheumatic fever. On closer examination, heart disease was
discovered in only 18 percent of the 93. Of the remainder
—those who did not have any heart abnormality—40 percent or 30 children were "restricted" in their activities. Six of
them were severely restricted, ostensibly because they had
heart disease. Most of the restrictions were imposed by
physicians, but parental zeal was a contributing factor. In
this case, therefore, the amount of disability resulting from
nondisease *exceeded* the disability due to actual heart disease.
Medicine caused more disability than it cured.[28]

Damage is done and disease caused by the medical care system for a number of reasons. There is no malice on the part of practitioners or administrators. The medical care system is subject to the same foibles, imperfections, and inefficiencies that plague all large institutions. One of the major differences, however, between the medical care system and many other large institutions lies in its capacity to do harm. An unavoidable conclusion is that the way in which our medical care system has evolved has created conditions that increase the likelihood of damage to patients.[29]

In *Medical Nemesis,*[30] Ivan Illich takes the argument to near extremes. He argues that medicine unquestionably injures more than it cures—not just through crude technology, but essentially because it has stripped patients of the tools to take care of themselves. Illich refers to this as "social iatrogenesis."

A medicine trapped in the logic of intervention with elimination of symptoms as its principal objective may act too hastily when the elimination of symptoms appears expedient, may ignore potentially untoward by-products of the means used to treat those symptoms, and, most deplorably, may fail to comprehend the lesson that thousands of deaths represent.

The Placebo: How Patients Get Less Than They Bargained For.   The placebo has a long and respected history. The use of chemically inert medications is common practice. In fact, until the last few decades, most medicinals were pharmacologically inert, and, in that sense, the "history of medical treatment until relatively recently is the history of the placebo effect."[31] But there is more to the placebo than pills. For example, one use of the placebo is in the treatment of warts. The healer paints the wart with a brightly colored but inert dye and instructs the patient that when the color has worn off, the wart will disappear. It works as often as any other treatment, including surgery.

Shamans and shamanistic ritual can be traced throughout

history. Contemporary analysts often discount shamans as healers because of their alleged use of chicanery. For example, a common technique among shamans is the use of blood-stained down, which is expelled from the mouth after "treatment." In many instances, no human tissue was or could have been extracted to "produce" the expectorate. But this is beside the point; since its importance was symbolic, this use of down is no different from the prescription of null medications. Jerome Frank, a psychiatrist at Johns Hopkins who has extensively examined the use of placebos, says of it:

> The most likely supposition is that it gains its potency through being a tangible symbol of the physician's role as a healer. In our society, the physician validates his power by prescribing medication, just as a shaman in a primitive tribe may validate his by spitting out a bit of bloodstained down at the proper moment.[32]

The placebo may be far more than a symbol. The expectations of some patients about a treatment can alter or even reverse the action of a pharmacological agent.[33] Frank recounts an experiment in which patients subjected to an emetic, an agent designed to cause convulsive stomach contractions and regurgitation, were told that their stomachs would not become upset. The subjects did indeed overcome the drug—they experienced no stomach discomfort.

When disease has a clear emotional base, the effectiveness of the placebo appears to be enhanced. In one study, patients with bleeding peptic ulcers were given a placebo but informed that it was a powerful and effective drug. Other patients were given the same agent but were advised that it was a new and promising experimental drug of undetermined effectiveness. The first group scored 75 percent in their remission rate; the second only 25 percent.[34]

The effectiveness of the placebo is not entirely understood, although it appears to be related to the "belief" of the patient in its efficacy. Thoughtful observers, like Frank, think there is more to it. The healer as well as the patient must believe in the efficacy of the treatment, or at least skillfully convey a state of belief to the patient. As Frank puts it:

> If the effectiveness of the placebo lies in its ability to mobilize the patient's expectancy of help, then it should work best with those patients who have favorable expectations from medicine and, in general, accept and respond to symbols of healing.[35]

To some patients the healer may be the most effective placebo. The placebo, whether a drug or some other treatment, may serve only as a material symbol of the healer's power.

The placebo effect demonstrates that medicine can cure some patients through its symbolic presence, simply by being there. But at what cost? If cures can be achieved by a fusion of the patient's belief in the treatment and the manifestation of symbols of healing, we must ask if it is possible to use equally effective but less expensive symbols.

Caring: How Patients Get Something But Not Necessarily What They Pay For. It is easy to be too scientific in condemning medicine. For centuries healers have administered to patients, with little impact if measured by the test of effectiveness. Until recently, medicine had few weapons. But medicine worked in the past and still works today, although with mixed results. Medicine has effective technologies— technologies that link what the physician does with what happens to the patient. But healing also occurs without sophisticated technology. A major ingredient has been "caring."

A number of research studies have assessed the Hawthorne effect. Most of the research was designed to ascertain optimal conditions for the production of goods. But the investigators discovered an anomaly—whatever they did,

production improved. The conclusion was inescapable.
When workers believed that management cared, whether by
increasing or decreasing the lighting, for example, they tried
harder.[36] Of course, there are limits; increasing the temperature in an office to an intolerable level may not be viewed as
caring. But the point is well-established—"caring" motivates
workers. It motivates patients as well. In fact, it may be
a determinative factor in healing. Some patients given
placebos respond better to the null "treatment" than those
given active drugs. In some studies, groups of patients given
placebos had better treatment outcomes than groups treated
with active medications.

Again Jerome Frank's analysis is pertinent. The symbols
of healing, unadorned with any proven technology, can
cure. One of the dangers, then, of too rigorous an examination of medicine—requiring proof beyond a reasonable
doubt—is that caring might be lost in the process.

THE IMPACT OF MEDICAL CARE
ON HEALTH STATUS

At the turn of the nineteenth century, an observer described
medical care in a way that still fits:

> There is a great difference between a good physician and a bad
> one; yet very little between a good one and none at all.[37]

Available evidence and underlying theory both indicate
that medical care has considerably less impact on health than
is generally assumed. Medical care is effective when applied
to certain illnesses. In procedures such as reduction of frac-
tures; treatment of infectious diseases such as diphtheria,
tetanus, poliomyelitis, and tuberculosis; and surgery for removal of pathenogenic organs, the physician truly heals.
Medical care also heals when it utilizes therapies with which

it has been entrusted. Penicillin, sulfa drugs, and antibiotics have expanded the capacity of the medical care system to treat and heal. But there remains much that medicine cannot do. Lewis Thomas, M.D., former Dean of the Yale University Medical School and now at the Sloan-Kettering Institute, says:

> The genuinely decisive technology of modern medicine is exemplified best by methods for immunization against diphtheria, pertussis, and various virus diseases and the contemporary use of antibiotics and chemotherapy for bacterial infections. The capacity to deal effectively with syphilis and tuberculosis represents a milestone in human endeavor, even though full use of this potential has not yet been made. And there are, of course, other examples: the treatment of endocrinologic disorders with appropriate hormones, the prevention of hemolytic disease of the newborn, the treatment and prevention of various nutritional disorders, and perhaps just around the corner, the management of Parkinsonism and sickle-cell anemia. There are other examples, and everyone will have his favorite candidate for the list, *but the truth is that there are not nearly as many as the public has been led to believe. . . .*[38]

It is commonly understood that medical care cannot cure cardiovascular disease, most cancers, arthritis, multiple sclerosis, stroke, advanced cirrhosis, and the common cold, to name a few. Of course, there are some exceptions. The Papanicolaou test for cervical cancer has proven utility,[39] and the means have been found to treat some forms of skin cancer. But cancers and heart disease cannot presently be cured.

Paradoxically, some diseases that are both preventable and treatable continue to strike large numbers of people. Allen Chase in *The Biological Imperatives*[40] lists a number of preventable diseases which either kill or debilitate large numbers of people simply because resources have not been allocated to their control. Included are hookworm disease, which afflicts approximately 600 million people; ascariasis, another worm infestation; schistosomiasis; trachoma, which causes irreversible blindness; and endemic goiter. The fact that most of these diseases are rampant in underdeveloped areas does not make them irrelevant.

Even in the United States there are diseases that could be more effectively treated, or possibly even prevented. An example is illness affecting the digestive system. According to Dr. J. Edward Berk, Chairman of the Department of Medicine at the University of California at Irvine, more than half of the population of the United States registers frequent complaints about digestion. Roughly 15 to 20 percent of all illnesses reported afflict the digestive tract—the stomach, intestines, biliary passages, liver, and pancreas.[41] The data are probably understated. Because of nonspecific symptoms, many cases of peptic ulcer and gallstones, for example, remain undetected. Nevertheless, digestive disease ranks second only to circulatory disorders as a cause of workdays lost per year. It ranks first as a cause of hospitalization.[42] Although digestive disease causes this much sickness, the number of gastroenterologists is inadequate, according to Dr. Berk. And research funds are disproportionately spent in other areas, particularly those that have strong lobbies, such as cystic fibrosis and muscular dystrophy.

Despite its limitations and despite its questionable priorities, the medical care system continues to grow and consume more and more resources. This is partly because we do not yet know enough about medicine's effectiveness. But we know some things—we are just beginning to ask the right questions. Some of the most trenchant thinking about the effectiveness of medical care has been done by A. L. Cochrane in his assessment of the British National Health Service. In *Effectiveness and Efficiency*,[43] Cochrane concludes that the National Health Service has had little to do with improving mortality and morbidity rates. He acknowledges the effectiveness of some medications for some conditions; strikes a loud note for preventive measures such as immunization and curtailment of population growth and cigarette smoking; expresses doubt about some tried and true measures, including the pap smear and the coronary care unit; and, almost hesitatingly, argues that further development of medical therapies should be deferred until definitive proof of their effectiveness is available. To read Cochrane is to conclude with him that little of medical care is effective and that health will never be the exclusive product of medical care—there are too many other factors.

When somebody gets the flu, the advice given by both the professional practitioner and the amateur diagnostician is the same—wait it out. A great deal of disease is self-limiting.[44] The human body, for reasons that are not completely understood, strives for equilibrium. This is the result of selective evolutionary pressures, which cut both ways. First, man can develop resistance to many diseases.[45] Tuberculosis is an example.[46] But, mysteriously, some diseases never strike some cultures at all. Several researchers have established the rarity of cancers, vascular disorders, and other degenerative diseases among primitive populations. As illustrated in Chapter 3, disease patterns vary greatly around the world. Unique geographical and cultural factors affect both the incidence and control of certain diseases.

In recent history, human beings adapted to new environmental conditions. In the nineteenth century, at the height of the Industrial Revolution, thousands of migrants were compressed into urban industrial sinks. Sickness and death resulted. But despite the human loss, enormous in some cases, people in most affluent countries have adopted to urban conditions (and, of course, the conditions have been improved as well). To use a concrete example, the devastating disease known as "consumption" in the nineteenth century is now understood to have been pulmonary tuberculosis. Although the virulence of the bacilli is as great now as it was then, our adaptive response has come to blunt its severity. In short, both the types of disease and the patterns of disease reflect prevalent conditions in a given culture. To quote René Dubos:

> Without question, nutritional and infectious diseases account for the largest percentage of morbidity and mortality in most underprivileged countries, especially in those just becoming industrialized. Undernutrition, protein deficiency, malaria, tuberculosis, infestation with worms, and a host of ill-defined gastrointestinal disorders are today the greatest killers in these countries, just as they used to be in the Western world one century ago. In contrast, the toll taken by malnutrition and infection decreases rapidly wherever and whenever the living standards improve, but other diseases then become more prevalent. In prosperous countries at the present time, heart diseases constitute the leading cause of death, with cancers in the second place, vascular lesions affecting the central nervous system in the third, and accidents in the fourth. Increasingly also, persons who are well fed and well sheltered suffer from a variety of chronic disorders, such as arthritis and allergies, that do not destroy life but often ruin it.[47]

The insignificance of medical care in improving health status cannot be overemphasized. Increased longevity, reductions in maternal and infant mortality, and other related improvements are not owed to medicine. Diseases associated with industrialization—largely infectious disorders—were tamed in developed cultures. The result was a steady improvement in health. But no new gains have been reported. If anything, due to our incapacity to adjust to the stresses of postindustrial society, health status is tapering. John Powles, in a paper on the ebbs and flows in health and disease patterns, summarizes the point:

> Industrial populations owe their current health standards to a pattern of ecological relationships which serves to reduce their vulnerability to death from infection and to a lesser extent to the capabilities of clinical medicine. Unfortunately, this new way of life, because it is so far removed from that to which man is adapted by evolution, has produced its own disease burden. These diseases of maladaption are, in many cases, increasing.[48]

Social factors are even more underrated than the environment. John Cassel, a noted epidemiologist at the University of North Carolina, has argued for more research focused on the relationship between disease rates and social phenomena such as industrialization, stress, and congestion. He points to the major shifts in disease patterns which have been portrayed and concludes:

> Despite intensive research, the explanation for the genesis of these changes in disease patterns have proved so far to be relatively unsatisfactory. . .[49]

The Comparative Impact of Other Factors on Health Status. It is a sad commentary on biomedical research that more attention has not been given to the *relative* impact on health of many variables, including medical care. It is generally agreed that contaminated food, degraded air and water, garbage and filth, and drafty, cold housing can cause illness. But the assumption has not been pinned down by research. Consequently, a reallocation of resources has not been undertaken. But there has been some work.

Economists have contributed more than their share. A 1969 study focused on the "production function" in health—its effectiveness in terms of what it is supposed to do. The study revealed that factors associated with income and education have a significant impact on health status.[50] The wealthier and more educated a person is, the healthier he is likely to be. Figure 1 illustrates the relationship between family income and health status. The effect of education on health was illustrated by a National Bureau of Economic Research study that examined interstate differential and age-adjusted death rates. One finding was that as large a reduction in mortality is associated with the expenditure of one more dollar for education as an additional dollar spent on medical care.[51] These findings have been dramatically corroborated by the Institute of Medicine of the National Academy of Sciences in a study that used anemia as a

FIGURE 1   HEALTH   STATUS   BY   FAMILY   INCOME—PERSONS
AGED 45–64

Family Income	Restricted Activity Days per Person per Year	Bed Disability Days per Person per Year	Work Loss Days Among Currently Employed Persons per Year	Percentage of Persons with One or More Chronic Conditions	
				Limitation in Amount or Kind of Major Activity	Unable to Carry On Major Activity
Under $3000	38.6	12.9	9.9	22.7	7.4
$3000–$3999	24.5	7.5	7.7	14.9	3.7
$4000–$6999	20.0	6.2	7.7	10.4	2.1
$7000–$9999	17.4	5.5	5.8	7.7	1.1
$10,000 and over	15.4	5.2	5.4	5.9	0.8

Source.   U.S. Department of Health, Education, and Welfare, Public Health
Service, *Age Patterns in Medical Care, Illness, and Disability, United States—July,
1963–June, 1965,* Series 10, no. 32, National Center for Health Statistics
(Washington, D.C.: U.S. Government Printing Office, 1966), tables 17 and
22.

"tracer" condition (a disease "followed" through the medical
care system to examine its detection and treatment in order
to generalize about the detection and treatment of other
conditions.) The study demonstrated that the education level
of the patients was more highly correlated with health than
with the source of medical care.[52] The study has to be read
carefully—all it demonstrated is that education is a proxy for
health; it correlates with health, but does not necessarily
cause it.

Another economist, Charles T. Stewart, Jr., has examined
the relative importance of different allocations of resources
to health. In comparing treatment, prevention, information,
and research, he found that both literacy (as a proxy for
information) and potable water (as a proxy for prevention)
had high impacts on life expectancy in all nations in the

Western hemisphere. Neither research nor treatment were significantly correlated. The data showed virtually the same results for the United States alone.[53]

Finally, the economist Eli Ginzberg, in *Men, Money, and Medicine*,[54] discussed the impact of nutrition on both physical and mental health. Ginzberg approvingly quotes an earlier report stressing the importance of nutrition for physical development:

> a diversified enriched diet will probably contribute to the health of the population . . . more than any other specific addition to medical resources, such as an increase in the number of doctors or the number of hospital beds.[55]

But Ginzberg points out, paradoxically, that "for the first time in our history more people die prematurely because they eat too much than too little."[56] This irony is reflected in other research as well. Victor Fuchs, in an unpublished paper, points out that affluence frequently leads to excessive consumption, even engorgement of some goods, such as rich foods, that adversely affect health.[57] Morbidity data reflect this well; the least healthy members of our population are white males over 55, the population cohort most likely to overconsume, overwork, and underrest.

A link between nutrition and health has also been established by studies contrasting the impact on health of nutrition and medical care. The sites were poor villages in the underdeveloped world. In one village, only improved medical care was introduced; in another, only nutrition was enriched; in a third, both medical care and diet were enhanced. The results show that nutrition was far more significant in improving health than the provision of medical care.[58]

Little cost-benefit or cost-effective research has been focused on the medical care system.[59] A few studies have assessed the relative benefits of selective disease control programs and maternal and child health care programs. In both cases the results, while tentative and crude, tend to prove the worth of certain disease detection programs. In general, programs that provide increased services for mothers and children in areas that have traditionally had few medical services have the greatest payoff. But, despite this, few low-cost, high-benefit programs have been established. Fluoridation programs, which are relatively inexpensive, produce benefits (in terms of reduced numbers of cavities) in more than 300,000 children for an expenditure of $10 million. Treatment-oriented programs for the same amount of money potentially benefit only 18,000 to 44,000 children.[60]

Little evidence of impact of mental health services exists. No cure is known for schizophrenia, the most prevalent psychosis, although proponents of megavitamin treatment profess to have had some success. The use of tranquilizers and shock therapy has also had some impact on reducing hospitalization rates. But rehospitalization rates are no better than with other therapies.[61] There are also claims for the effective treatment of depression. The overall record is mixed at best.

There is, however, some evidence that social and environmental factors may play a role. In *Mental Health,* a series of epidemiologic studies are reviewed.[62] The factors purportedly related to mental health included poor housing, congestion, poverty, and nutritional deficiencies. Although not all the studies confirm the hypothesis of the authors, the conclusion is reached that two of the studies "suggest strongly that improvement in social environment probably does have a favorable effect on mental health."[63]

There is a hard issue here. The fact that treatment is emphasized over prevention is not entirely the fault of medicine. In the case of maternal and child health, fluoridation programs, and other similar programs, the choice of whether to fund or not to fund is a political

decision. In this sense the choice of treatment over prevention can be said to be a choice made by the public. But, given
the power and mystique of medicine, it is also true that the
public's choices about health matters are strongly influenced
by physicians and, to a lesser extent, other health professionals. Medicine has chosen treatment over prevention, and
it continues to defend its choice. Prevention programs are
starved at least in part because medicine wants too much of
the loaf. But the problem cannot be camouflaged by making
medicine the only villain. Prevention programs are also
starved because medical care is often a "life and death"
matter. No arguments and no logic will convince terrified
parents that the resources needed to treat their child would
be more rationally allocated to prevention. This is a major
reason why prevention programs are crippled. Medicine
could do far more to inform public opinion, but the problem
would remain. This is why I argue, in some detail later, that
our basic conceptions about health must change if medicine
is to change. The public's value preferences are real; only
when those value preferences change will medicine change.

In combination, then, the empirical evidence and the
theory seem convincing; medical care has a limited impact
on health and is most effective when applied to certain
identifiable conditions where there is evidence about its effectiveness. But when contrasted with all the other factors
that demonstrably affect health, medicine plays a minor role,
despite being cast for lead.

3

Medicine: A.D. 1974

Medicine started out a poacher. It simply incorporated measures that seemed to work. But even at its pragmatic best, there were doubts. Oliver Wendell Holmes, Sr., wrote in 1860:

> Throw out opium, which the Creator himself seems to prescribe, for we often see the scarlet poppy growing in the cornfields, as if it were foreseen that whatever there is to be fed there must also be pain to be soothed; throw out a few specifics which our doctor's art did not discover; throw out wine, which is a food, and the vapors which produce the miracle of anesthesia—and I firmly believe that if the whole *materia medica*, as now used, could be sunk to the bottom of the sea, it would be all the better for mankind—and all the worse for the fishes.[1]

The history of medicine reflects the constant interplay of art and science. The Hippocratic era established the scientific foundation of medicine four centuries before the Christian era. But all early medical systems blended the scientific with strong doses of mystique. The empirical side of medicine manifested a healthy respect for common but strikingly pragmatic practices. As Lord Ritchie-Calder observed about Assyro-Babylonian medicine of roughly 2000 B.C.:

> For example, sore eyes were, and are still, common in lands of the khamsin, the hot dry wind which blows out of the Arabian

desert. The eye trouble was ascribed to the Demon of the Southwest wind, the image for which was a dog-headed eagle with lion's claws. The wind was supposed to be frightened by the ugliness of his own image, which, accordingly, was set up outside the houses to keep him and his afflictions away. To treat sore eyes, the priest-doctor would prescribe cutting up an onion and mixing it and drinking it with beer. This was obviously to encourage tears, with (as we now know) their germicidal properties. Then the eyes were to be assuaged with oil.[2]

But sound empirical observations were often accompanied by repugnant rituals. Calder continues:

So far this is commendable treatment but, by priestly reckoning, not drastic enough against such a nasty demon. So to the straight-forward prescription was added the ritualistic one: "Thou shalt disembowel a yellow frog, mix its gall in curd and apply to the eye."[3]

Medicine is a very different undertaking today. It is durably wedded to the scientific method, frequently to the detriment of the "art" in medicine. How did medicine get this way?

THE EVOLUTION OF THE EXISTING
MEDICAL CARE SYSTEM

Four Traditional Dualities.   Medicine can be characterized by four dualities that persist today. The first is reliance on both empirical investigation and magic. Shamans performed theatrical stunts to summon spiritual support for their crude but often effective therapies. The Asclepian medical tradition, drawn from Greco-Roman history, also exemplifies this duality. Physicians trained in this tradition not only utilized drugs and some surgical techniques, but also invoked the gods to assist in the cure.

In the centuries to follow, the interplay between empirics

and art continued—horseback riding as a therapy for digestive disorders was common as late as the mid-nineteenth
century. For practitioners who possessed some competence
in both, the mixture of art and science probably worked. But
when plied by practitioners with neither skill, or with only
one of the two, it seems to have been disastrous.

Medicine finally yielded to the "logic" of the scientific
method as it passed into this century. A sage physician has
observed that "somewhere between 1910 and 1912 in this
country, a random patient, with a random disease, consult-
ing a doctor chosen at random had, for the first time in the
history of mankind, a better than fifty-fifty chance of
profiting from the encounter."[4] Until 50 years ago, few truly
effective therapies were known. Care consisted largely of
prolonged nursing-home stays and the alleviation of those
symptoms amenable to the few weapons medicine possessed.
Just over a hundred years ago, only half the children born in
the United States reached their fifth year.

Hospitals, so integral to medical care today, were virtually
unknown until the late 1800s. Medical technology had no
need for specialized facilities—the black bag was more than
sufficient. Hospitals were not needed until medicine became
mass-produced, until convenience to the doctor became
more important than the welfare of the patient. Today hospitals are little more than inefficient factories with elaborate
safety rules. The early practitioner could manage his patients with bedside manners, a few nostrums, some salves
and balms, and a few tools.[5]

The hospital was also a product of an era of institution
building. Hospitals were built at roughly the same time that
prisons were first constructed, and when schools became
fortresses instead of simple one-room learning experiences.
The need for institutions to house "problems" probably
emerged during the same time—society wanted prisons to
lock up and treat deviants, schools to baby-sit, and hospitals
to produce and sell health more efficiently.[6]

The second duality arises from the contrasts between individual medicine and population medicine. Modern medicine focuses on the individual. The division between medicine and public health occurred early in this century, at about the time medicine became infatuated with the scientific method. Today, schools of public health stress the prevention of disease in populations; schools of medicine, reflecting a curative bias, educate physicians to treat the symptoms of ill health in individuals. Unfortunately, the two types of training seldom overlap. Kerr White, a medical care researcher at Johns Hopkins University, refers to the early twentieth century division of medicine and public health this way:

> The drive to improve medicine cure to the neglect of medicine care carried the day. Flexner's views prevailed and the "basic" sciences of medical education were declared to be biochemistry and physiology; the equally "fundamental" sciences of epidemiology, economics and sociology were excluded from the curriculum. In spite of the pathologist Virchow's admonition that medicine is essentially a social science, America opted for individual medicine largely to the exclusion of population medicine. . . . Population medicine was relegated to so-called schools of public health after World War I.[7]

The schism between population medicine and individual medicine, aside from being a historical anomaly and a tragic mistake, may have been unavoidable. Population medicine is not a saleable commodity. A community may suffer from disease, but a community, as distinguished from an individual, lacks the cohesiveness to purchase its health. Individual medicine, conversely, taps a potent market; to many, health is worth nearly any cost. But the costs and consequences of the schism are becoming clearer. There is no synergy in medical care. The care of some does not necessarily result in a healthier whole.

The third duality is attributable to a philosopher rather than to a physician. Medicine (among other things) has been greatly affected by the Cartesian division between mental and physical states. The Hippocratic tradition emphasized the interrelationship between body and mind, but the Cartesian influence on medicine resulted in separate physical and mental health service systems. The training of a physician treats physical states in mechanistic terms and mental states in cursory terms, and thus drives a wedge between them. To use René Dubos's words, "instead of attempting the hopeless task of understanding man as a whole, scientists have felt free to deal seriatim with the various aspects of man's nature."[8] Once medicine had divided the body and mind and chosen the body as its focus, it was only a small step to equate the working of the human organism with the precision of machine function. The apotheosis of physics and chemistry after Newton led biology into frenzied comparisons between living things and machines.[9] Medicine followed suit.

The error implicit in the division between mind and body is now being recognized. Our growing understanding of our bodies, nourished by information about the interconnectedness of humanity with the rest of nature, is slowly leading to a more "holistic" theory of health. But at the same time, a powerful paradigm in mental health has appeared, and this paradigm, Skinnerian behaviorism, is a direct descendant of the mechanistic paradigm of the physics and chemistry of the past. William Irwin Thompson makes the point this way:

> [I]n our physical sciences we have long since gone beyond the 18th century notion of dead hunks of matter moving in the black void of space. Yet, our psychological sciences are still restricted to 18th century mechanistic notions: minds are simply . . . hunks of grey matter moving in the black void of time.[10]

The fourth duality arises in the physician's psyche. The relationship of physicians to patients has always been somewhat schizoid. Historically, physicians functioned not only as

healers, but also as counselors, confidants, and friends, roles
that display the anthropological side of medicine. But with
the advent of new and more sophisticated medical hardware,
and the specialization that characterizes today's medicine,
the technical aspects of the physician's practice are emphasized. Many physicians still dispense homely wisdom and
act as friends and counselors to patients. But specialization
and assembly-line processing of patients has become inevitable. The patient can no longer be treated as a whole person
because few physicians are equipped to do so.

The relative importance of the technical and anthropological aspects of care has been controversial in medicine. But
the proponents of technical medicine have had the better of
the argument, and as a result have dramatically influenced
the evolution, nature, and style of the medical care system.
However, the argument is far from over; neither is it an
either/or question. Proponents of anthropologic practice do
not argue that medical technology has not contributed (and
cannot contribute) to the quality of care. What they emphasize is the profound importance of the "texture" of the
relationship between physician and patient, which can
influence the health of the patient.

Although the issue is not yet resolved, all sides to the
debate agree that change, and particularly change in the
relationship between healer and patient, is possible only if
both the role and the function of the physician is transformed. Michael G. Michaelson, a critic of the medical care
enterprise, suggests a direction for change:

In the wake of radical technological and societal change our
idea of "doctor" remains rooted in the nineteenth century
model. Today's physician is perhaps the last remaining ar-
chetypal American—a self-sufficient, independent, rugged individual after the frontier model, with illusions of omniscience
and (not only as he controls the allocation of health resources
on a national level) a life-style of omnipotence. It is impossible
to understand the pathology of American medical education

and care without first understanding the essential obsolescence
of the American physician. And it is only on the basis of this
understanding that the fundamental restructuring of American medicine . . . can amount to anything more than the
"patchwork approach."[11]

Present Trends. All four dualities are present today. A few
physicians rely on the "arts" of medicine, but most surround
themselves with gadgetry and insulate themselves from the
pains and passions of their patients. Biomedical technology,
fruit of the scientific pursuit of health, has solved only a few
of the puzzles of disease. And modern medicine has yet to
find an appropriate mix of preventive and curative regimens. Writing in the *AMA News* as recently as 1972, Dr.
Russell Roth, then the speaker of the American Medical
Association's House of Delegates, expressed medicine's view
of preventive care by characterizing the role of the physician
as "almost by definition, one of sickness care."[12]

Although there is a growing appreciation of a "holistic"
approach to patient care, medicine is far from achieving that
goal and, given evolutionary constraints, is unlikely to get
there. Dubos points out a few of the constraints:

> The holistic approach, however, corresponds to an abstract
> ideal not amenable to full achievement in practice either by the
> clinician or the public health officer. Most medical situations
> are so complex that their determinants can never be ap-
> prehended in all their details; it is impossible consequently to
> deal with them only on the basis of scientific knowledge.[13]

In the last few decades, medicine has experienced a flood
of technological development, spurred by heavy investment
in biomedical research and development, advances in the
basic sciences, and refinements in electronic instrumentation
and computerization. One result is that the physicians have
become purveyors of extraordinarily complex wares. Patients who present problems amenable to new techniques are

now the preferred targets; for example, some physicians who seek to make history through transplantation of vital organs may assay their patients for donors.

Until technology made specialization possible, physicians were generalists, utilizing a range of techniques with varying degrees of complexity. Today, at least half the physicians in this country are specialists.[14] Many physicians specialize so that they will be presented with manageable and finite health problems to which they can can apply the most elegant techniques available. Medicine has become and is constantly becoming more and more reductionist in its approach. The Hippocratic tradition has been splintered. Each of the four dualities reduces the patient to a more simple set of properties.

This, then, is the paradox: Medicine aspires to perfection, even miniaturization—reduction of the patient's problems to manageable and manipulable sets. But as it does so, it erodes its capacity to deal with the health of the people, despite its claims that it does so. Eliot Freidson, a medical sociologist, agrees when he says, "The Medical profession has first claim to . . . the label of illness and *anything* to which it may be attached, irrespective of its capacity to deal with it effectively."[15]

Moreover, as is increasingly clear, because medicine has failed to encourage the patient to assume the responsibility for health, the public craves more and more services, however specialized and fragmented. The public has been convinced that human suffering is a disease that medicine can cure. People are less willing to accept pain. They are shrill in their denial of suffering, and enervated by their dread of death. Medicine has become a synonym for health when it can do little more than modulate human suffering. Although estimates vary, well over one-half of those who seek physician's services do not have medical disorders. Rather, they are afflicted by disorders of the spirit bred by the suffering and anguish that accompany life. And yet, tragically, even sophisticated twentieth century medical techniques can do little to heal these afflictions. Nevertheless, medicine has fostered a profoundly dependent public which searches for cures that do not exist.

ORGANIZATION, PRACTICE, AND STYLE

Organization and Structure. The medical care industry has often been called a "cottage industry." This does not mean that sophisticated technology has not been used, but rather that the way in which the system is organized remains almost feudal in nature. Kerr White observes:

> The health care industry today is about at the same stage of development as the railroad industry was after World War II. With the physicians and hospitals in control, it is a near industrial monopoly. It has a complacent administrative style and a large, cumbersome and self-serving regulatory mechanism that does not encourage or even accommodate change.[16]

Medical care is still largely provided by solo practitioners in their offices, or by institutions, including hospitals and nursing homes, that are influenced and often controlled by practitioners. But despite their control of hospitals, few physicians have entered into formal arrangements with hospitals; they are usually treated as independent contractors. Occasionally, of course, doctors and hospitals join to provide services, but in such cases there is no powerful centripetal force.

The result is that the industry has remained both labor intensive and highly fragmented, despite rapid technological advances.[17] Many different medical care services are provided by an array of health practitioners and institutions, including doctors, hospitals, clinics, visiting nurses, laboratories, drugstores, and pharmacists. And the physicians, who have the power to tie things together, function independently of one another, relying on informal communication and referral practices.

The more than 7000 hospitals in the United States differ greatly in size and technical capacity. Regardless of size, each possesses only two basic ways to deal with patients—they are either placed in a bed or treated as outpatients. Hospitals are designed primarily for the care of bedridden patients. Physicians and consumers alike tend to think of and use hospitals for the care of acute conditions requiring immobilization, and for chronically ill patients who are often housed in hospitals because there are few other places to put them.

As a result, outpatient facilities have been shortchanged. They are neglected by everyone, patients included. It is easier for physicians to manage patients who are confined to bed. Moreover, many patients, particularly when someone else is paying, prefer the attention they get while in a bed to standing around unnoticed in the outpatient department. Hospitals and other facilities for care rarely reflect the fact that patients' conditions range along a continuum from well-being to mortality; not every condition can be classified as insubstantial or acute.

The Distribution of Medical Care Resources. Four interrelated problems affect the distribution of medical care resources in the United States: the location of resources, patients' ability to pay for medical care, patient access to care, and specialization of physicians.

First, medical care resources are spatially maldistributed along two dimensions: rich/poor and urban/rural. The more affluent states average 160 practicing physicians per 100,000 people, almost double the rate of 87 physicians per 100,000 in the less affluent states.[18] And despite heavy population concentrations in major metropolitan areas, and high physician to population ratios in most standard metropolitan statistical areas (SMSA), few of the poor have easy access to care. The fact that the poor average as many visits to the doctor as the nonpoor is only testimony to their persistence.[19]

Patients' ability to pay for medical care relates to the rich/poor dimension, but not necessarily in spatial terms. Many of the poor and near poor in this country lack care because they cannot pay for it. Since Medicaid only aids those who are among the poorest, many low-income families are without care, no matter where they live. Although many physicians continue in the tradition of treating patients who cannot pay, Medicaid undercuts the physician's incentive to provide charity care. The effect of Medicaid, then, has only been ameliorative—not curative. The Medicaid program attacked the consumer's purchasing power problem by augmenting the capacity of the poor to pay, but stopped short in two crucial respects. First, it does not cover all the health needs of those eligible for its support; second, it aids only the very poor. The near poor and beleaguered middle-income consumers are left on their own.

The patient access problem, although closely related to it, is more complex than the problem of the geographic distribution of physicians. The local availability of physicians is, of course, a necessary precondition to access. But many persons residing in areas that provide medical care resources still do not have access to care, because they do not know where to go or what to do. Some may recall the halcyon days when the family doctor came to call. But the house call disappeared years ago, along with the family practitioner. Today many persons do not know a healer of general competence, or even anyone to advise them where to go or what to do. More than 50 percent of patient visits to emergency rooms do not involve emergencies; people go there because they do not know where else to go. Recent studies have pegged the level of nonemergency use of emergency rooms even higher—in one case at 90 percent. And the volume of demand has greatly increased in recent years. In one study, the percentage of nonemergency visits rose from 45.4 percent in 1960 to 72.5 percent in 1967.[20] These data depict a public that does not know where to go when illness strikes.

The fourth problem—the distribution of physicians by specialty—has a significant effect on overall distribution, since the type of medical care available may be as important as the overall quality of services available. The trend toward specialization among physicians is unmistakable. In 1970, the American Medical Association formally recognized 29 new specialties, which brought the total to 63. At present, roughly 55 percent of all physicians in the United States deal with primary care (general practitioners, internists, obstetricians, and pediatricians). Only 21 percent classify themselves as "general practitioners." If current trends continue, the percentage of primary care physicians will drop to approximately 50 percent by 1980.[21]

Specialization by physicians aggravates the distribution problem by reinforcing the tendency of physicians to practice in affluent urban areas rather than in rural and poor areas. Specialists need to practice where the population is concentrated to insure a sufficient number of patients for their services.

In sum, then, the maldistribution of medical care resources is a compound of too few health care resources in sparsely populated areas, too few health care resources in heavily populated urban/poor areas, constraints on access to care in both rural and urban areas because of consumers' inability to pay, and the lack of access to primary care practitioners, assuming the presence of such practitioners. And all of these problems are in turn compounded by the increasing specialization of physicians.

Control of Performance.   A predominant characteristic of the medical care system is the pervasive role played by professional societies and associations of providers. There are many illustrations.

- State laws grant the "right to practice" only to physicians who procure licenses and, through the same means, circumscribe the activities of other health professionals and paraprofessionals.
- The boards responsible for the issuance of licenses are controlled, in some cases exclusively, by professionals.
- Regulation of hospitals through hospital facility licensure, accreditation programs, and training program approval is similarly either controlled by providers or effectively subject to their control.
- Review of the quality of care, when undertaken, is conducted only by physicians through peer and utilization review committees, "tissue" committees, and mortality conference committees.
- Physicians fix the employment patterns and size of the labor market in health, and although they are not specialists in management, insist on filling the multiple roles of director, advisor, and technician.
- The distribution of health manpower by specialty, and spatially by location of practice, is largely determined by the availability of training and practice opportunities, which are also controlled by providers.

We now have a thoroughly professionalized medical care system. More than 100,000 individual "firms" of professionals render care to a bewildered public. The system is formidable and confusing at the point of entry, swathed in mystique during the treatment process, and aloof and obdurate about its results. We pay an enormous price to perpetuate the system, most of which goes to the salaries of highly paid professionals and the amortization of the mortgages on our hospitals. We let the professionals allocate resources and determine the distribution of facilities. Physicians deploy themselves as they please. And, to a large extent, the number of hospital beds is constrained only by the limits of capital and imagination. Finally, we have made no attempt to judge the system's product—physicians insist on the right to monitor the performance of the system by standards of their own making.

The behavior of the existing medical care system is intimately related to prerogatives of professionals. Eliot Freidson, in *Professional Dominance*,[22] offers some reasons:

1. Professionalism rests on a body of arcane knowledge. Thus, questions about efficacy are met with disdain; it is the province of professionals to make independent judgments.

2. A "lock" on information is critical to preservation of professional mystique. Freidson argues that the "prime reason for the failure to communicate with the patient does not lie in underfinancing, understaffing or bureaucratization. Rather it lies in the professional organization of the hospital and in the professional's concept of his relation to his clients."[23]

3. Professionals reserve to themselves the right to regulate their performance. This is at the heart of the concept of professional autonomy.

4. Medical professionals in particular, since they emphasize that the importance of what they do is not to be questioned, argue that the cost of what they do is similarly not to be questioned.

5. Physicians make nearly all of the work rules by which other personnel within the medical care system are governed. They set the tone for the administration and behavior of the entire system.

6. Professionals prize knowledge and the specialized application of that knowledge. Proliferating specialization in medicine and the emphasis on high style practice are two results.

The shape and nature of the medical care system is the result of many factors. But woven throughout is the unmistakable, if often immeasurable, influence of the physician.

Many physicians acknowledge that most disease is self-limiting. In many instances all the physician can do is diagnose, prescribe, and then instruct the patient to take over. But most patients do not know how to take over. Some manage for themselves and others with home care. Some measures undertaken at home work; others probably do not. This, of course, is also true of care in the hospital. But most home care measures have not been tested against medical care in the hospital. When they have, home care has not suffered by comparison, even in the treatment of acute conditions.

In one study conducted in England, for example, the treatment of acute myocardial infarction—heart attack—was as efficacious to the patient at home as hospital-based treatment.[24] But since few studies of this sort have been conducted, and since this study conflicts with another, we do not know which is better—sophisticated care in the hospital, home care, or some mixture of both. Perhaps when we have more information, both approaches to care can be utilized, the choice or mixture dependent on the nature of the problem and the patient's attitude. But it is the patient's attitude that is the most problematic.

The Expanding Scope of Medicine. Today few patients have the confidence to care for themselves. The inexorable professionalization of medicine, together with reverence for the scientific method, have invested practitioners with sacrosanct powers, and correspondingly vitiated the responsibility of the rest of us for our health. Medicine has deeply penetrated society. Many judgments made by medical practitioners are heavily freighted with moral considerations. A growing list of social "problems," including aging, drug use and addiction, alcoholism, pregnancy, and genetic counseling, have been or are becoming "medicalized."

These problems, with the possible exception of genetic

counseling, have customarily been regarded as either natural processes or human weaknesses, not as "diseases." But today, alcoholism is often no longer a crime, but a sickness to be treated. And pregnancy, for centuries a natural process maturing and reaching its termination outside the hospital without medical supervision, is now almost wholly subject to medical management.

Irving K. Zola, a sociologist at Brandeis, argues, "The list of daily activities to which health can be related is ever growing and with the current operating perspective of medicine seems infinitely expandable."[25] This occurs, in part, because many customary activities, like drinking, sex, and even eating are subject to social standards. And as individuals fail to meet society's standards, their deviance is translated into illness. David Mechanic, another medical sociologist, characterizes the "medicalization" of certain behaviors this way:

> The traditional approach . . . seeks to identify an underlying disorder . . . that explains the apparent deviant manifestations, and thus introduced into the medical model, these behavioral syndromes are increasingly identified as diseases.[26]

Zola marshals some convincing data. "Clinical entities," or potential disease indicators, occur in 50 to 80 percent of the population examined in health surveys or by periodic checkups. But even more astonishing is the degree to which society has become "medicalized" through drug use. Zola refers to a recent study showing that within a 24 to 36 hour period, from 50 to 80 percent of the adult population in the United States and the United Kingdom takes a prescribed or "medical" drug.[27]

The fundamental point of Zola's analysis—medicalization—is the result of another point he discusses: the relationship between the expansion of medicine and the "dependency" of patients. By creating dependence, medicine has yoked patients to its cart. Zola argues that one of the principal reasons for this is the "capture" of many of the common activities of life by medicine, and their concomitant transformation into "medical problems." In part this has occurred because medical institutions, like other institutions, have sought to ensure their survival through growth. But, as Zola argues, another reason why medicine has sought to expand its franchise lies in its recognition that many diseases are caused by behavior that lies beyond its reach. Zola points out that many physicians, for example, feel that a change in diet may be the most effective treatment for a number of cardiovascular disorders and perhaps some cancers. Physicians have had little control over the food preferences of their patients; but this may change. Zola alludes to an article in *Time* magazine that captures the mood, entitled "To Save the Heart: Diet by Decree."[28]

Recognition by doctors of the salient causes of illness is welcome. Medicine should not necessarily be pilloried for seeking to "treat" more problems if it possesses the tools to help. But it rarely does—it cannot cure alcoholism. Medicine may not be the best agent to treat human failings; there may be other and more effective approaches. Nevertheless, one thing is clear. The expansion of medicine raises a dilemma: As medicine encroaches on more of human life, it further incapacitates its major ally—the patient—from assuming responsibility for health. In so doing, it weakens its own capacities to heal.

Of course, medicine is only one case in point. Fragmentation, specialization, and a divergence between the goals of professionals and clients characterize all professional services today. But what is tragic is not what has happened to the revered professions, but what has happened to us as a result of professional dominance. In times of inordinate complexity and stress we have been made a profoundly dependent people. Most of us have lost the ability to take care of ourselves. We have been progressively stripped of the skills and tools to do so. Our bodies are the cannon fodder of a reductionist, mechanistic medicine. Our emotional lives are buffeted by the fear that our behavior will subject us to the ministrations of mental health professionals. And our practical business and work worlds are increasingly governed by obfuscating legal terminology and practitioners.

NATIONAL AND TRANSNATIONAL CONSIDERATIONS

Historically, health has been a national undertaking. This has been true whether medical services have been a responsibility of central government or assumed by local government with measures of private charity. The twentieth century has seen the "nationalization" of health services in the Western hemisphere.[29] The trend toward centralization of health services has, however, been accompanied by a wide range of delivery financing and regulatory alternatives. In some countries, such as Sweden and Great Britain, health services have been nationalized;[30] in other countries, such as France, elements of the private sector remain.[31] In the United States, the private sector has remained virtually intact but is heavily subsidized through public third-party payment programs such as Medicare and Medicaid, and may, with the passage of a national health insurance plan, become almost totally subsidized.

But questions of health transcend national boundaries. Current concerns with allocation of resources and increased mobility and information have begun to internationalize our concepts of health.

Resources, Health, and National Boundaries. The United States consumes roughly 35 percent of the world's electrical power. Although other nations have not matched our gargantuan appetite, it is nevertheless true that the more developed the nation, the more likely it is to consume a disproportionate share of world resources. Under such circumstances, the demands of less developed nations for more of the resource "pie" will become more strident. Resolving these demands without armed conflict will necessitate a reordering of priorities by all nations. Among the priorities to be scrutinized will be expenditures for medical care.

Within a few years, it is likely that health services in the United States will absorb 9 percent of gross national product; currently, they consume nearly 8 percent,[32] a figure topped by some nations. The percentage of GNP devoted to health represents a substantial portion of the national wealth of all nations.[33] It is unrealistic to assume, in the interest of equity alone, that developed nations will unilaterally pare medical expenditures and transfer resources to less developed nations. However, it may not be unrealistic to achieve economies of size through consolidation of elements of delivery systems among nations.

Multinational corporate activity appears irreversible.[34] Corporate development at the transnational level results in conflicting allegiances and responsibilities on the part of multinational bodies. Individual nations find it difficult to regulate effectively corporate bodies that transcend national boundaries. Thus, increases in transnational activity will inevitably lead to demands on the part of multinational corporations for transnational status (but not necessarily regulation). Affected nations will need to establish regulatory mechanisms. In fact, world organizations may be needed to control the continued development of multinational corporations.

The rise of multinational corporations suggests the need for more sophisticated world health organizations, as well. Employees of multinational corporations, because of their high mobility, will in effect become men and women without a country. Historically, health services have been paid for and received in the country of domicile. The erosion of domicile may result in the corporate employer assuming (or being compelled to assume) the responsibility for the provision and financing of medical care services for its peripatetic employees.

Finally, with more trade, more multinational corporate activity, more public and quasi-public transnational development, and with accelerated dispersal of people throughout the world, the rapid "transmission" of disease agents from country to country is inevitable. Under such circumstances, a world health organization will have to be established to facilitate international disease control.[35]

The case is fairly clear. Health problems do transcend national boundaries, as do many other nagging problems such as air and water pollution, sanitation, and even education. But some nations have developed more sophisticated responses than others. In the United States, medical care has reached a degree of sophistication vastly greater than in most other nations, and probably superior to any other country. Its only rivals are Sweden, Great Britain, and a few other countries. One might argue, then, that what the United States has should be exported. But there is more to it than that.

Variations in the Incidence of Disease. Cancer is found everywhere in the world. But marked disparities exist in the incidence of certain types of cancer among populations. For example:

- Hepatic cancer is prevalent in Africa and Southeast Asia, Indonesia, Java, and Sumatra. In these countries, hepatic cancer accounts for as much as 80 percent of all cancers recorded. In most Western countries, the rate is less than 2 percent.
- Cancer of the stomach disproportionately afflicts the Japanese, a large part of Western Europe, and northern South America. Nearly half the cancers in Japan

are in the stomach. In comparison, in Southeast Asia
and in parts of Africa the incidence of stomach cancer
is infinitesimal.

• Cancer of the lung, pleura, and bronchi is highly prevalent among males in Western Europe, the United
States, and Australia. Little or no lung cancer has been
reported in Korea, Ceylon, India, Burma, and
Trinidad.

• Cancer of the uterine cervix is relatively pronounced in
India and China, but less prevalent in Western Europe,
the United States, and Australia.[36]

Disparities are also observable in the rates of infectious
diseases. Although some of the differences may be due to
lack of prevention programs, infections are far more frequent and more severe in passage from the temperate zone,
through the Mediterranean, to the Tropics. Diseases such as
smallpox and typhoid are found nearly everywhere; diseases
such as trachoma, schistosomiasis, yellow fever, and plague
are specific to geographic areas.

Disparities in disease rates also exist among various countries within the same geographic zones. Poliomyelitis, for
example, is more prevalent in the temperate zone, but un-
explained variations in rates of the disease from country to
country in that zone have been recorded. In 1949, the cases
reported per 100,000 were 413 in Iceland, 37 in Sweden, 14
in England, 2 in Belgium, and 1.1 in Yugoslavia.[37]

Another dimension of variation can be shown through
longitudinal examination of disease patterns. In general, the
so-called "diseases of civilization" afflict persons in the more
highly developed countries such as the United States,
whereas the infectious diseases continue to decimate populations in less developed countries. But the impact of infectious diseases was substantial in the United States some
decades ago when the level of development in this country
was roughly comparable to that of nations now classified as

underdeveloped. A World Health Organization survey, conducted to elicit expressions of major health problems for the year 1963–64 and answered by 147 governments listing 46 problems, showed that the problems varied according to regions. Figure 2 depicts the regional profiles of health problems and, by implication, their relationship to developmental stages.

The varieties of diseases and the variation in disease rates are arguments for the maintenance of domestic medical care systems. Countries must tailor the provision of medical care services to the needs of their populations. But it is a matter of degree. We will fail to understand the variations in disease both within countries (since countries are at various developmental stages) and among countries if a world health viewpoint is not encouraged.

Delivery System Development.   Although medical care services are much alike, differences exist between delivery system arrangements among various countries. The differences are great between highly developed countries with sophisticated delivery systems and less developed countries with rudimentary systems. Nevertheless, a review of the history of the organization of medical services reveals a convergence among the systems. Increasingly, where the direct provision of services has not been assumed by the central government, the financing of care and its regulation (in countries where there is a private sector) have become more centralized. For example, in the United States the medical care system is still largely private, but enactment of a national health insurance plan will accelerate the centralization of medical care. Such a program will bring our medical care system closer to the systems of other advanced Western nations, such as Sweden and Great Britain, even though a national health insurance scheme is not the same as the national health services of those countries. A national health insurance scheme under-

FIGURE 2 REGIONAL PROFILES OF HEALTH PROBLEMS

Major health concerns	Africa	Western Pacific	Southeast Asia	Americas and Caribbean	Eastern Mediterranean	Europe	Australia New Zealand Japan	Canada United States
	28	27	7	34	14	20	3	2
Malaria	○19	○8	○3	○10	○2		○1	
Tuberculosis	○17	○24	○3		○10	○11		
Leprosy	○9	○11	○2					
Helminthiasis	○9							
Bilharziasis	○9							
Diarrhea and dysentery	○9	○9	○7	○13	○7			
Filariasis		○8	○3					
Deficiencies in organization and administration	○6		○1	○5	○7	○12		○1
Trypanosomiasis	○6							
Onchocerciasis	○5							
Venereal disease	○6	○12		○13		○9	○1	○2
Malnutrition	○6	○6	○3	○16	○3			
Environmental deficiencies	○5	○11	○7	○13		○11	○3	
Smallpox	○3		○2					
Cholera (including El Tor)		○6	○2					
Meningitis	○1 – 2							
Yaws	○1 – 2							
Enteric fevers	○1 – 2							
Trochoma	○1 – 2		○2		○6		○1	
Infectious hepatitous	○1 – 2					○11		○1
Accidents	○1 – 2					○6	○3	○2
Respiratory virus diseases		○5				○11		
Population pressure		○5	○3					
Cancer				○2		○9	○3	○2
Chronic degenerative disease				○4	○3	○9	○3	○2
Alcoholism				○4			○1	
Movement of people					○5			
Urban congestion					○1			
Vascular disease of central nervous system							○1	
Mental disorders				○4		○6	○3	○1
Narcotics						○1		
Dental health		○4				○1		○2
Indigenous population						○1		
Aged and chronically ill								○1
School health								○1
Handicapped								○1
Manpower								○1

writes the cost of care provided by private practitioners and hospitals. In a national health service, most practitioners and hospitals are absorbed into a public system.

The convergence of medical care systems lessens pluralism in the provision of care. Medical care systems, as they have evolved, reflect unique social, cultural, and disease conditions within countries. In many cases, they also meet political imperatives within those countries. As delivery systems become more alike, however, their autonomy is undermined.

Equity and Human Development. In the *Asian Drama: An Inquiry into the Poverty of Nations,*[38] Gunnar Myrdal hammers home the point that health cannot be considered in isolation from other elements in the development process. Myrdal argues that health both affects and is affected by other socioeconomic factors, including income, life styles, and nutrition. For example, Myrdal believes that health and education are highly interdependent. A child's ability to benefit from schooling depends on the child's health, and an adult's ability to utilize the knowledge and skills acquired through education depends on mental or physical fitness. Reforms in health, then, are necessarily social reforms.

Myrdal also emphasizes the importance of integrating

Source. John Bryant, *Health and the Developing World* (Ithaca, N.Y.: Cornell University Press, 1969), Figure 3. Developed from a questionnaire reported by the World Health Organization in *Third Report on the World Health Situation, 1961–1964,* No. 155 (Geneva, 1967), pp. 28–35. Some data were taken from a prepublication mimeographed document of the same title. Used by permission of Cornell University Press.

Notes. The figure at the top of each column indicates the number of countries reporting. Circles and figures in columns indicate the number of countries listing the particular health problem as a major concern; a black circle indicates regional consensus that the problem was one of the most important. The vertical line arbitrarily separates less developed from more developed regions. The horizontal line separates diseases of greatest concern to less developed regions from those of greatest concern to more developed regions.

health with other socioeconomic institutional and policy
initiatives:

> From the planning point of view the effect of any particular
> policy measure in the health field depends on all other policy
> measures and is, by itself, indeterminant. This means that it is
> impossible to impute to any single measure or set of measures
> a definite return in terms of improved health conditions. A
> generalizable model, in aggregate financial terms, visualizing a
> sum of inputs of preventive and curative measures giving rise
> to an output of health conditions cannot be of any help in
> planning. In fact, such a model presupposes the solution of the
> planning problem, for it is premised on an optimum combina-
> tion of all policy measures, which cannot be achieved without
> taking account of circular causation within the health field and
> in the whole social system.[39]

The blunt fact is that the failure to provide health to
populations in less developed countries means simply that
those countries will not develop. It would be draconian to
assume that the more developed nations are not concerned
about the less developed world. But it would be naive to
assume that the more developed countries will voluntarily
divest themselves of resources to accelerate the development
of the less developed nations. So it is still a matter of equity.
Is there any justification for the expenditure of thousands of
dollars to maintain the health of an American, when for the
same amount of money the afflictions of hundreds and even
thousands of people in less developed countries could be
ameliorated?

Thirty million people die of starvation alone every year—
one every second. Schistosomiasis, cholera, malaria, and
diarrhea can be curbed and in many cases eliminated. The
technology to control these diseases is known. Nonetheless,
millions of people suffer and die from them. In the United
States, thousands of dollars are spent to install one cardiovascular care unit for treatment of myocardial infarction—a disease more common in highly developed
countries—with less than spectacular results.

Figure 3 makes the case poignantly. John Bryant writes that this figure:

> shows the causes which contribute substantially to the deaths which are in excess of those expected if rates among young children were at the level of the rates in the United States. Deaths from diarrheal diseases account for an estimated 179,000 deaths or 17 percent of those in the age group under five years in Latin America. The expected number, based on U.S. rates, would be only 3,500, and an excess of 175,000 results, which is 22 percent of the total excess from all causes.

FIGURE 3 ESTIMATED DEATHS UNDER FIVE YEARS OF AGE IN LATIN AMERICA FROM SELECTED CAUSES IN 1969 AND EXPECTED DEATHS ON BASIS OF RATES IN THE UNITED STATES

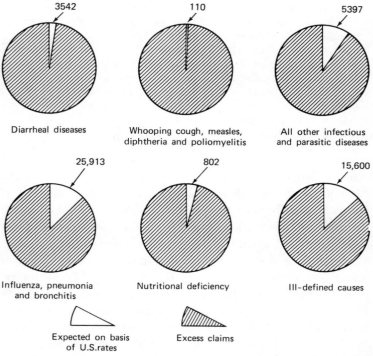

Source. John Bryant, *Health and the Developing World* (Ithaca, N.Y.: Cornell University Press, 1969), p. 45. Used by permission of Cornell University Press.

The deaths from measles, whooping cough, diphtheria and poliomyelitis, preventable through immunization, caused an estimated 57,000 deaths in 1969. If death rates from these causes had been at the U.S. level, only 170 deaths would have occurred. Excess deaths from all infectious and parasitic diseases form 36 percent of the total excess. Deaths assigned to nutritional deficiencies as the underlying cause totalled 22,959 compared to the expected number of 802. Acute respiratory diseases—influenza, pneumonia, and bronchitis—were designated as the cause of 217,000 deaths. The expected number would be 27,000 and the excess 190,000. A large group of deaths in Latin America fall into the ill-defined group, mainly because of lack of medical attention prior to death.

Clearly, child health must remain at the center of health plans for the coming decade. Progress has been made, but much more is required to prevent needless morbidity and mortality. Techniques are now available for prevention of many of the communicable diseases of childhood, which cause excessive mortality in Latin America. Environmental sanitation programs will also contribute to reductions in mortality from some of the infectious diseases, especially diarrheal diseases. However, attention must be directed to associated causes and conditions. For example, malnutrition, which is not adequately described by morbidity and mortality statistics, plays a leading role in high child mortality when occurring together with infectious or respiratory diseases.[40]

As a further example, in 1963 throughout the world 124,000 deaths, mostly of small children, were attributed to diarrhea. Deaths due to diarrhea in the United States are virtually unknown. The burden of the disease falls most heavily on children in less developed countries. In Colombia, 92 percent of the deaths due to diarrhea are in children under five. But diarrhea is only one cause of child mortality. In the United States, children under five represent roughly 10 percent of the population and account for somewhat less than 7 percent of all deaths. In less developed countries such as Thailand, Jamaica, and Guatemala, children under five represent, on the average, approximately 17 percent of the total population, and account for 35 to 60 percent of all deaths.[41]

There may be geopolitical reasons for the vast disparities in the resources brought to bear on the diseases that afflict people from country to country, but the unalterable fact is that disease in a human condition, and that its cure should transcend politics.

Although the case for equity can be strongly made, a simple reallocation of medical care resources alone will not overcome the economic deficiencies of the less developed nations. The medical care services gap will probably never be completely closed, but it can be narrowed.

The solution to problems of development transcends the shifting of medical care resources. Even if the most developed nations, such as the United States and most Western European nations, were to divert resources otherwise available to them for medical care services to the less developed nations, it is unlikely that the developmental level of those nations would be significantly improved. In 1965 the GNP per capita in the United States was $3600. In Indonesia the GNP per capita was $99. Based on then prevailing population and growth rates, it will take Indonesia 593 years to reach the U.S. GNP per capita.

Staggering disparities are also found at the level of per capita health expenditures. Both Nigeria and Jamaica allocate more than 10 percent of all government expenditures to health, which is more than the United States on the basis of GNP, but on a per capita basis this amounts to 40¢ in Nigeria and $9.60 in Jamaica. Nigeria could spend its entire governmental budget on health, but on a per capita basis its expenditure would not equal Jamaica's.[42] Some of these variations are illustrated in Figure 4.

The case is made even more starkly in Figure 5. The figure illustrates the number of years needed for selected developing nations to reach the U.S. GNP per capita level of $3600 based on the year 1965.

There are many reasons why the organization of medical services should be undertaken at the international level. But despite the logic of the case, there are some problems; in

FIGURE 4 TRENDS IN GOVERNMENTAL EXPENDITURE ON HEALTH SERVICES, SELECTED COUNTRIES

Country	Fiscal Year	(1) General Government Health Expenditure (Capital and Current) (mills.)[a]	(2) (1) as % GNP	(3) (1) as % General Government Expenditure	(1) in Terms of Expenditure per Inhabitant Local Currency	U.S. $
Kenya	1956–1957	£2.2	1.0	4.7	0.3	0.8
	1962–1963	3.4	1.3	6.0	0.4	1.1
(% change)[b]		(+54.5)	(+30.0)	(+27.7)		
Tanzania[c]	1958–1959	£2.2	1.2	9.8	0.2	0.7
	1964–1965	3.4	1.3	9.2	0.3	0.9
(% change)[b]		(+54.5)	(+4.8)	(−9.4)		
Colombia	1958	Pesos 161.0	0.8	6.6	11.9	1.4
	1964	533.0	1.0	11.0	30.5	3.5
(% change)[b]		(+231.9)	(+29.1)	(+66.6)		
Chile	1957	Esc. 51.3	2.3	11.6	7.2	9.3
	1963	241.8	2.5	11.1	29.4	13.7
(% change)[b]		(+372.0)	(+8.8)	(−3.7)		
Thailand	1957–1958	Baht 102.0	0.2	1.6	4.1	0.2
	1963–1964	352.0	0.5	3.4	11.9	0.6
(% change)[b]		(+245.1)	(+110.0)	(+112.5)		
Indonesia	1957–1958	Rph. 721.0		2.9	8.2	0.3
	1963–1964	6404.0		2.8	64.0	0.2
(% change)[b]		(+788.2)		(−3.4)		
United States[d]	1957–1958	$5364.0	1.2	4.1	30.4	30.4
	1963–1964	9034.0	1.5	4.7	47.4	47.4
(% change)[b]		(+68.4)	(+21.7)	(+14.6)		

58

Source. John Bryant, *Health and the Developing World* (Ithaca, N.Y.: Cornell University Press, 1969), Table 9. A partial reconstruction of a table in World Health Organization, Official Records, *Third Report on the World Health Situation, 1961–1964*, No. 155 (Geneva, 1967), pp. 52–53. Used by permission of Cornell University Press.

[a] Includes all governments, institutions, and agencies, whether central, intermediate (state, provincial, regional, etc.), or local. See WHO, *Third Report*, pp. 52–53, for further definitions.

[b] Any apparent discrepancies in the percentage changes shown are due to the rounding of their constituents for presentation in this table.

[c] Former Tanganyika only.

[d] In the U.S., about 25 percent of the expenditure for health services is from governmental sources, the remainder from private sources. Total per capita expenditure for health services was about $200 in 1964 and has since increased substantially.

FIGURE 5   YEARS NEEDED TO ACHIEVE CURRENT U.S. GNP PER CAPITA

	1965 GNP per Capita (1965 U.S. $)	Number of Years Needed to Reach $3600 per Capita[a]
Sweden	$2497	11
Canada	2464	12
West Germany	1905	16
East Germany	1574	17
France	1924	18
United Kingdom	1804	19
Czechoslovakia	1554	20
Japan	857	22
Israel	1334	24
Australia	2009	25
USSR	1288	28
Italy	1101	30
Poland	962	34
Romania	757	38
New Zealand	1932	42
Argentina	492	69
Taiwan	221	71
UAR	166	97
Thailand	126	98
China	98	101
South Africa and South West Africa	503	115
India	99	117
Brazil	280	130
Pakistan	91	144
Mexico	455	162
Nigeria	83	339
Colombia	277	358
Indonesia	99	593

Source. Herman Kahn and Anthony J. Wiener, *The Year 2000: A Framework for Speculation on the Next Thirty-Three Years* (reprinted with permission of the Macmillan Company; © by the Hudson Institute, Inc., 1967), p. 149.

[a] The number of years needed to reach $3600 per capita was calculated on the basis of the 1965 GNP for each country and the "medium" rate we projected for growth of population and GNP. The "numbers of years needed" is thus simply a way of looking at the *rate* at which the country's GNP per capita seems likely to approach the current U.S. level in the "standard world"; obviously, to the extent that the "number of years" is large, many factors can be expected to change in the interim.

particular, three problems are posed for the United States. First, there will be pressure on the United States to share its resources. It would be naive to assume that the United States will do much about it, but the fact remains that the resources consumed in this country for medical care would have a far greater payoff in other parts of the world, particularly because of the inextricable link between health and development.

At the same time, the "limits" of medical care are being reached in the United States. Thus, the second problem lies in the nature of modern medicine. The sustained growth and development of a "services" approach to health throughout the world will bankrupt treasuries everywhere. The cost explosion in the United States threatens the public purse. And the British Health Service is near to bankruptcy, because, contrary to the predictions of the architects of the service, demand for services in Great Britain has not subsided.

The demand has not abated because illness has not abated. Medical care alone cannot produce health. Brian Abel-Smith, in his international study of health expenditures, has shown that there is no correlation between the level of medical expenditures and identifiable needs for health care—the richer countries spend more absolutely and in relation to total resources.[43] Some medical services are essential, but the full panoply of services available in the United States are not needed elsewhere and may never be.

The hard question, then, is whether the shift from a medical "services" approach to the "promotion" of health can be made before, or at least when, the limits of "services" are reached, or whether the appetite of medicine will outstrip the capacity of nations to promote health through a variety of measures, including medical care. The issue will undoubtedly first arise in the United States, where evidence is surfacing that medical care is no longer engendering health. But it seems inevitable nonetheless that the United States will be asked to "export" services and medical technology—the very services and technology that may constrain the evolution of a wiser and more effective approach to health in receiving countries.

If the underdeveloped world is to have health, it must not blindly emulate the United States; it must not import a medicine designed to treat patients whose illness arises from their impoverishment, and whose sickness is a condition of existence.

One more problem remains. As long as the American public spends more on chewing gum than on social services, what difference does it make that inequities and inanities characterize the international allocation of resources? Should we not remedy things at home first? There are two responses. First, attacking one inequity does not preclude attacking another. Second, the future lies in internationalism. Most national solutions are anachronisms, even if they are necessary in the short run. So in the design of a new medicine, a task taken up in the last chapter, the international context must be considered.

THE VARIETIES OF MEDICINE

Dr. Frances Crick, the British biologist who shared a 1962 Nobel Prize for the discovery of DNA, has said:

> Americans have a peculiar illusion that life is a disease which has to be cured. . . . Everyone gets unpleasant diseases and everyone dies at one time. I guess they are trying to make life safe for senility.[44]

Crick isolated a critical premise of Western, or allopathic medicine—that disease has to be cured. But allopathic theory and medicine is only one approach to health—a disease-oriented approach. Because allopathic medicine has "selected" only some phenomena for investigation, its vision and tools are limited. A variety of other approaches to healing can be taken. Acupuncture is one of them.

Figure 6 is a reproduction of fingerprints photographed by Thelma Moss and Kendall Johnson, who are conducting research on radiation photography at the Neuropsychiatric Institute at the University of California at Los Angeles.[45] Radiation photography depicts the "energy field" around the body. This field apparently varies in relation to certain stimuli, including bodily manipulations or interventions, and possibly with thought processes. This "field" has also been referred to as the "field of mind."[46]

Emerging field theory may illuminate acupuncture medicine. According to acupuncture theory, energy in the body courses through specific points along bodily meridians. In a healthy organism, the "energy" flow is unimpeded and accordingly the body is in a state of equilibrium. However, if the energy flow becomes blocked, or promiscuously released, acupuncture—the insertion of needles at various acupuncture points—can be utilized to reestablish equilibrium. Through the reestablishment of equilibrium, acupuncture apparently alters the body's energy field. In Figure 6, the picture on the left depicts a fingerprint in its normal state. The picture on the right shows the same finger after an acupuncture needle had been inserted in the subject's upper arm and left there for 5 minutes.

FIGURE 6   NORMAL FINGERPRINT (*left*) AND FINGERPRINT AFTER ACUPUNCTURE

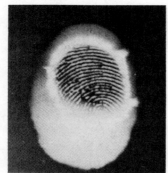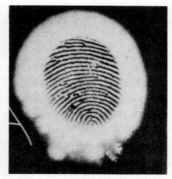

Source. Harper's Magazine, January 1973. Used by permission of Thelma Moss, Ph.D.

Radiation photography does not "prove" anything; the process is still in its infancy. It seems clear that the human body is surrounded by a "field," but we do not fully appreciate the significance of the heightening in the body's energy field that results from acupuncture. There is evidence that acupuncture works, however, and we can assume that its efficacy might be related to its effect on the body's energy field.

The purpose of this illustration, then, and of the other illustrations in this section, is not to demonstrate that allopathic medicine is wrong, but rather that it is fallible. The work of Johnson and Moss with radiation photography suggests that there is a "life" or "energy field" surrounding the human body. This fact alone, if convincingly established, will not repudiate allopathic theory. But it will be evidence that there is a newly discovered phenomenon—the energy field—which might serve as an indicator for use in diagnosis and healing.[47] There are healers who base their practices on body field or aura readings.[48] Some healers claim that a person's aura or field alters with the presence of disease, and that therapy has as its purpose the restoration of the natural field.

The dispute about acupuncture is now in full fire. Reports about its effectiveness, principally as an anesthetic agent, proliferate. There no longer is much doubt that it works —doubts are only expressed about how it works. This is ironic, since there is no generally accepted theory of anesthesia in allopathic practice. Andrew Weil, a physician and drug researcher, describes the anomaly:

> although anesthesia has been around for over a hundred years and although millions of persons have been put into the state under close observation, no satisfactory theory of general anesthesia exists; doctors have no idea what these drugs do to the brain that accounts for the state.[49]

What underlies the skepticism about acupuncture? In part, it is attributable to the inflexibility of allopathic practice, its intolerance of inconsistencies. This is not surprising since all paradigms—and allopathy is a rigid paradigm —elicit extraordinary loyalty. But in part it is also a perceptual problem. In tests performed at the Menninger Clinic in Kansas, Chief Rolling Thunder, a Shoshone medicine man, was asked to "cure" a contusion on a subject's leg. The Chief employed one of his favorite methods. He placed his mouth over and around the bruise, sucked vigorously, then dashed to the opposite side of the room and vomited. The bruise disappeared at roughly the same time that the scientists in the room rushed to retrieve the vomitus.

To the scientists, the "cure" could only have been effected if the damaged tissue in the bruised leg had somehow been physically extracted. Of course, it was not removed in the sense in which the scientists could have understood it. But the bruise disappeared. And the explanation probably lies in perception. To the subject and the Chief, the sucking and the vomiting were elements of drama underpinning a belief system—a belief that a cure could be achieved. To the observers, the material substance, the vomitus, was the key. The two groups perceived the episode differently, and the explanation for the cure may lie in this perceptual difference.[50]

An example drawn from acupuncture practice might clarify the point. Acupuncture practice is inconsistent with Western medical theory in several ways. To begin with, for an operation to be performed on any part of the anatomy, acupuncture needles may be placed in different parts of the body for different patients. In one hospital the needles might be inserted into the forearms, while in a second, the placement points might be the neck and the ankles. According to the allopathic theory of pain—the specificity theory —this makes no sense. Under allopathic theory, specific points in the body receive and transmit signals to the brain. The theory dictates that the person will experience pain precisely at the point of the stimulus. In contrast, acupuncture theory is nonspecific. Two universal forces, the yin and the yang, both active in the body, must be in a state of balance. When disharmonies arise between the two forces, disease and pain result. The yin and yang flow through the body along roughly 12 meridians. Acupuncture insertion points—some 365—are deployed along these meridians. The manipulation of acupuncture needles is designed to restore harmony to the body.[51]

There are other medical theories and practices that are even at greater variance with allopathy. In both 1971 and 1972, the American Academy of Parapsychology and Medicine sponsored interdisciplinary symposiums respectively entitled "The Varieties of Healing Experiences: Exploring Psychic Phenomena and Healing,"[52] and "The Dimensions of Healing: A Symposium."[53] The conference reports contain articles that reflect recent research in paranormal and esoteric methods of healing. Two of the more fascinating, but problematic, reports feature Arigo, a natural healer from Brazil, who is now dead; and bodily control manifested by the Swami Rama, an Indian yogi who demonstrated his yogic training program under carefully controlled laboratory conditions at the Menninger Foundation clinics.

Arigo, an uneducated natural healer, saw thousands of patients in the course of his work. According to reports of his practice, he achieved striking results. His greatest strength was diagnosis. His diagnostic skills were carefully measured against diagnosis rendered for the same patients by allopathic physicians, and compared well with them. Arigo generated his diagnosis without the use of sophisticated technology, largely on the basis of visual scans of a patient. Although he utilized some modern techniques such as drugs, and occasionally performed surgery, his repertoire also included surgical repair without the use of any equipment.[54]

Swami Rama, under laboratory conditions at the Menninger Clinic, was able to generate electroencephalographic brain waves at will. Under similarly controlled conditions, the Swami also demonstrated his ability to stop his heart from beating. After he was "wired" for the demonstration and told to proceed, the electrocardiograph records reflected an increase in heart rate from 70 beats per minute to about 300 per minute. The experimenters had expected the heart rate to stop altogether and thus thought that the experiment had been a failure. However, when the EKG records were examined, the case appeared to be one of "atrial flutter," a state in which the heart fires at high speed without blood either filling the chambers or the valves working properly. The Swami had emptied his heart of blood, but it had continued to tremble. After a final examination of the records, the investigators concluded that the Swami had stopped his heart for at least 17 seconds. The Swami also "created" lumps like cysts in his muscles.[55]

The demonstrations by the Swami are extreme examples of biofeedback techniques, to use the Western term. The growing literature on biofeedback contains unmistakable implications for self-care.[56] Robert Ornstein, in his book *The Psychology of Consciousness,* devotes a section to some of the implications for medicine:

> As each new drug is developed, as each new surgical procedure is perfected, less and less responsibility for the cure is delegated to the patient himself. Although we have achieved an extraordinary amount of sophistication in drug and surgical therapy in western medicine, this development has been a bit unbalanced. We have almost forgotten that it is possible for the "patients" *themselves* to learn directly to lower their blood pressure, to slow or speed their heart, to relax at will.[57]

Ornstein then discusses the research of Johan Stoyva and Thomas Budzynski at the University of Colorado Medical Center. Stoyva and Budzynski have been investigating the use of biofeedback to "decondition" or "desensitize." If the patient can be taught through biofeedback to "learn" to

relax in situations normally associated with tension and
stress, phobias, headaches, and even anxiety itself might be
minimized.[58] Biofeedback demonstrates that the barrier between mind and body is permeable. If an individual can be
trained to exercise control over some bodily functions, self-
healing and self-restoration are possible. Furthermore,
biofeedback is not a skill peculiar to just a few persons. The
evidence assembled thus far suggests that everyone can
"learn" to exercise some degree of control. And the techniques are very simple and extremely inexpensive.

One of the most puzzling phenomena is Philippine
"psychic surgery." A number of uneducated healers clustered near Manila have purportedly performed "healings"
that entirely confound allopathic theory and most other
healing regimes as well. There are some written reports of
this method, and a few films.[59] The gist of the method is
simple but nearly incomprehensible to the Western mind.
The psychic surgeon appears to perform surgery without
instruments and can, in certain instances, penetrate the body
wall with his hands. The film I have seen, to be com-
prehended, requires a major widening of perceptual gates.
There are explanations of the practice based on theories
relating to the "astral" or "spirit" body. These are ill-defined
concepts, but they are in the same family of concepts as the
"energy" field or "field of mind" theories. I return to this
subject later, to discuss how the efficacy of the surgery, if
there is any, is related to the patient's and the healer's *belief*
in its efficacy.

Other examples can be drawn from more conventional
annals. Jerome Frank in *Persuasion and Healing*,[60] a thoughtful and provocative examination of the arts of healing, includes many illustrations. At Lourdes, for example, millions
have sought and some have experienced cures. Frank also
devotes attention to the healing power of shamans, particularly in the American Indian tradition.

Adherents of yoga and meditation have also advanced

arguments for the use of these practices in healing. Studies examining the physiological impact of Hatha yoga reveal that yoga practitioners experience weight loss; significantly improve their respiratory functions, principally through lowered rates of respiration; increase their vital capacity and breath-holding ability; and develop resistance to physical stress.[61] The impact of yoga on health has even led to a medicine based on yogic practices. Steven Brena, M.D., relates its basic tenets in *Yoga and Medicine*.[62]

A case for meditation has also been made—more efficient respiration, less stress, diminished use of drugs, alcohol, and stimulants, and so on.[63] Meditation has also found its way into medical care. Dr. Carl Simonton has made efficacious use of meditative techniques in the treatment of cancer patients. His technique is disarmingly simple. Simonton first teaches his patients how to meditate and then instructs them about their disease process and the means by which the body's natural immunities resist the cancer. He then asks them to meditate on the disease process and the "attack" on the disease by the immune system. It sounds simplistic and perhaps it is, but according to Simonton, for those patients who use meditation the prognosis is roughly twice as favorable as it is for another patient population matched for demographics, severity of disease, and attitude.[64]

The way medicine is practiced in the United States is commonly assumed to be not only the most scientifically pure way, but also the only way in which medicine can legitimately be practiced. Based on the historical record this is a false assumption. There are many medical theories and many varieties of medical practice.[65] Again, medicine in China illustrates the point. Prior to the nineteenth century, a traditional system of medicine was exclusively practiced in China. This system relied heavily on herbal medicine and acupuncture. In the nineteenth century, Western medicine was introduced to China by missionary doctors who founded both medical schools and hospitals on the Western medical model. Over ensuing decades the two systems of medicine competed for the loyalty of both the government and patients. Today, both systems of medicine practice side by side—it is called "walking on two legs" by the Chinese. The Western model is superior in surgical technique, in achievement of hygienic conditions, and in the treatment of infectious diseases that respond to antibiotics. Chinese practice is more efficacious in the treatment of diseases that are chronic, degenerative, and psychosomatic; precisely those diseases that are the least affected by medical practice in this country.[66]

Whatever the theory, there seems to be a constant: The most effective healers are time and self-help. The most reflective healers, whether physicians, natural healers, or chiropractors, acknowledge this. All the healer can do is to diagnose and then create the conditions, the climate, in which healing can take place. But healing requires belief in its efficacy. Modern medicine has systematically shorn its consumers of belief in their recuperative powers. It has fostered a pervasive and pitiable dependency. This is why healers operating outside traditional American medicine have always had a marginal but formidable claim upon the loyalty of many of those who are ill.

The effectiveness of nonallopathic healing undoubtedly varies as much as the effectiveness of modern medical practice, and certainly relies on skills. The need for competence does not vanish outside of modern medicine. An acupuncturist must possess a finely calibrated skill to "read" a patient's body; knowledge of 365 acupuncture points and a sensitivity to some 12 different bodily pulses, or meridians, each with 27 gradations, is required. This can be contrasted with the simple heart pulse rate and blood pressure readings taken by the physician, but only in number and kind of readings. Leaving aside efficacy, which can be debated endlessly (and in the absence of hard comparative data, seldom demonstrated), acupuncture in the hands of the skilled practitioner is considerably more complicated than much of modern medical practice. At the same time, a raw recruit to acupuncture may possess only a limited amount of information and even less skill.

Nonallopathic healing cannot be imperiously dismissed as charlatanism. The range of competence and skill among such practitioners, as with allopathic healers, is no doubt vast. A chiropractor who seeks to cure a patient's back pain by jumping heels first onto the patient's back is not necessarily a quack, but may be a well-intentioned bungler. Yet even on the basis of anecdotal information, the healing powers of many such practitioners are unmistakable, even if in need of further study. It is only a commentary on the medical care research establishment that we do not know more.

In many instances, medicine has refused to acknowledge the healing power of unconventional methods. The therapies originated by F. M. Alexander are one example.[67] The techniques developed by Alexander center on restriction of musculature. Some of the results include reductions in high blood pressure, increases in mental alertness and regularity and strength of respiration, and alleviation of circulation deficiencies. The efficacy of the therapy has been attested to by many commentators.[68] An account of Alexander's techniques is found in an article by Nobel prize-winner Nikolaas Tinbergen, "Ethology and Stress Disease."[69] Tinbergen refers to Alexander's work as a clear example of medicine's refusal to incorporate therapies with power effectiveness simply because these therapies do not fit conventional categories.

There is an irreducible element that distinguishes natural healing from the treatments and blandishments of modern medical care. The natural healer, whether physician or shaman, fosters and builds upon the confidence and belief of his patients. This is a crucial difference. Today's physicians create a climate of uncertainty and dependence and are consequently left with only the tools of massive intervention to effect a cure. Patients' complicity is seldom encouraged. Thus the most fundamental factor in healing is denied. Medicine neither takes patients where they are, as a whole, nor inculcates trust in their natural resiliency. In practice it dictates profound intervention since natural re- cuperation is neither fostered nor, because tools and train- ing dictate practice, sufficiently perceived. Natural healers, possibly less skilled and occasionally charlatans, construct their cure on the preexisting belief of the patient in the efficacy of the methods used. In short, they intuit and trig- ger the patient's will to be healthy.

Modern medicine has successfully isolated and denigrated nonallopathic practitioners and practice. But as more people turn to other strains of healing, as often as not because of the failure of modern medicine to heal them, the pressure on medicine to adapt will intensify. Evidence of the efficacy of acupuncture alone has focused the attention of consum- ers on the richness of other traditions of healing, and on the parochialism, if not impoverishment, of our indigenous practice.

BIOMEDICAL RESEARCH: THE SEARCH FOR CURES

For 1974, the federal government allocated $1,781,334,000 for health-related research.[70] The bulk of the money was allocated for biomedical research—research directed toward improving the physician's ability to treat and cure. Of the remainder, roughly $70 million was expended to improve the service capability of the medical care delivery system. To those who feel that this is a vast sum of money, medical care researchers point out that vastly greater sums are spent for national defense and security. Although a substantial dispar- ity exists between defense and health expenditures, there is also a fundamental similarity: Both spend too much money for the wrong thing. Defense spending is concentrated on war instead of peace, and health expenditures on cures instead of prevention.

Ever since Senator Matthew Neely luridly portrayed the ravages of cancer in 1928, a continuing theme in public policy has been the defeat of disease through research. Senator Neely used some memorable phrases:

> Mr. President, the concluding chapter of *A Tale of Two Cities* contains a vivid description of the guillotine, the most efficacious mechanical destroyer of human life that brutal and blood-thirsty man has ever invented.
>
> But through all the years the victims of the guillotine have been limited to a few hundred thousands of the people of France.
>
> I propose to speak of a monster that is more insatiable than the guillotine; more destructive to life and health and happiness than the World War, more irresistible than the mightiest army that ever marched to battle; more terrifying than any other scourge that has ever threatened the existence of the human race. The monster of which I speak has infested and still infests every inhabited country; it has preyed and still preys upon every nation; it has fed and feasted and fattened . . . on the flesh and blood and brains and bones of men and women and children in every land. The sighs and sobs and shrieks that it has exhorted from perishing humanity would, if they were tangible things, make a mountain. The tears that it has wrung from weeping women's eyes would make an ocean. The blood that it has shed would redden every wave that rolls on every sea. The name of this loathsome, deadly and insatiable monster is "cancer."[71]

The issue of a cancer cure had not lost its allure by 1971. Mary Lasker, a patron of the medical arts, entered to up-stage the late Senator Neely with these memorable phrases:

> Senator, you and the members of the U.S. Senate have the opportunity, if I may say so, seldom given in the lives of men—even Senators—to turn on the power that eventually

could save the lives of hundreds of thousands of men, women
and children in the United States and pass on that knowledge
all over the world, and the name of America would be blessed.

You and I have known some of your ablest colleagues who
might have been saved and the many dear ones in our own
families who still can be saved if we waste no more time and let
S. 34 be our next "man on the moon."[72]

Of course, cancer has not been the only target, even if it is
the next "moon shot." Other dread targets include afflictions
of the heart, liver, eye, and other organs; arthritis; and
sickness in children, mothers, and the psyche. Each has
elicited a suitable response. The National Institutes of
Health and Mental Health were created to channel public
support into health-related research.

There is little question about the "benefits" that have resulted from the cumulative expenditures over the years.
Countless numbers of scientists have improved and honed
the techniques of treatment. Among their successes are the
control of infectious diseases and the limitations of deaths
due to tuberculosis and pneumonia.[73] But there is a clinker.
The overwhelming emphasis in biomedical research has
been on the cure of disease, *not* its prevention. This is not
surprising. The two major influences that shaped the federal
research program had their stakes in cures, not health. The
first, a loosely knit but powerful consortium of private citizens, committees, and foundations, has fervently lobbied
Congress to spend money to find cures for diseases. This
lobby was fueled by the already sick and by relatives and
friends of the already dead. What good was prevention to
those who were sick and to those who have suffered the
anguish of the death of someone who had been "incurably"
sick?

The second major influence was medicine itself. When
Congress was willing to listen to appeals for research monies,
medicine was already yoked to the curative cart. The schools
of public health had been exiled from the mainstream of

medicine and surgeons were running the show then, as they do now. Prevention, then as theoretically profound as now, was an anathema—the money was needed for cures; prevention was a possibility when everyone was cured. Congress bought the line and is still buying it. The "War Against Cancer" is an enlightening case history.

The dialectic between the Congress, the Executive, and the powerful health lobbies is a fascinating illustration of the clash between rhetoric and reality. Stephen P. Strickland chronicles the struggle in *Politics, Science, and Dread Disease*.[74] Although they differed on tactics, the relentlessness of the lobbies and the "motherhood" nature of the issue combined to make the cancer crusade inevitable. Cancer is second only to heart disease as a killer. Estimates in 1973 pegged the death rate at 350,000, augured the discovery of 665,000 new cases, and predicted the treatment of 1,035,000 more.[75] But for more than a few reasons, the conquest of cancer is unlikely to be as successful as the conquest of the moon.

First, there are doubters. Dr. Salvador E. Luria, head of MIT's new cancer center, insists that "any vision of a crash program promising a 'cancer cure' in three, five, or ten years would be a self-delusion and a dangerous misleading of the public."[76] Agreeing with Dr. Luria, but moonstruck with the rhetoric surrounding the "Conquest of Cancer Act," Dr. Sol Spiegelman, Director of Columbia University's Institute of Cancer Research, argues that "an all-out effort at this time would be like trying to land a man on the moon without knowing Newton's laws of gravity."[77]

The second reason is technical. Cancer is not a single disease but a family of disorders. There are three prominent types of cancers: carcinomas, sarcomas, and more generalized forms such as leukemia and lymphatic diseases —multiple myelomas. And cancer is promiscuous in its choice of a site within the body—it can occur almost anywhere, although it varies in both incidence and virulence. A few cancers can be readily treated, but others are resistant to

treatment, and still others intractable and even refractory.
The diffusion of cancers and their variability of response to
treatment suggests a complex, even kaleidoscopic agent. If
this is true, there is no simple cure for cancer; there are only
cures for cancers. The conquest of cancer then is not like the
moon shot, but rather like multiple landings on the planets
of the solar system.

The third reason is the most important, but it is surprisingly simple. Assume that cures were discovered for all cancers, or at least that cures were discovered that protracted
life more than a few months. Would the problem of cancer
be solved? No. Cancer would simply be added to the list of
degenerative diseases which eviscerate life and the living and
hasten a certain death, but do not suddenly kill. The difference is like dying instantly in an automobile crash, or having
life chipped away with a dull hatchet. But despite this, the
rationale for the pursuit of a cure is that we do not know
what the cause is. But that claim—that we do not know the
"cause" of cancer—is simply wrong.

First, because there are many cancers, not one cancer,
there are *causes,* not a cause. And we do know some of them
even if we cannot identify them all. Cancer is a contemporary disease of contemporary life. It affects people differently depending on their geography, culture, and life style.
In the United States, cancer strikes hard in the breast, lung,
and colon. In Japan the stomach is the target. In Africa the
malignancies of the civilized world are rare, but lymphatic
disorders are common, along with cancer of the mouth.[78]

Cancer is a product of how people live; but people can live
differently. We have scores of leads on specific causative
factors: cigarettes and foul air "cause" lung cancer. Poor
penile hygiene probably "causes" most cervical cancer. An
array of known carcinogens in the air, in water, and in our
food can be linked with certain cancers.[79] Yet we persist in
trying to cure, to the neglect of research focused on prevention. If we know that the inhalation or ingestion of certain

materials and matter is linked with cancer, why is research not focused on behavioral changes, substitutes for dangerous products, and sociocultural engineering to minimize the risks? The reason is simple and absurd: those are not medical matters. Medicine only treats and cures. Someone else is responsible for the causes. The cause is important only to the extent it makes the cure possible. It is exactly like bombing the village to save it.

The budget of the National Institute of Cancer does contain allocations for "prevention," approaching in magnitude allocations for curative treatment. But the budgetary terminology is misleading. The word "prevention" has been badly treated. Prevention to the physician means seeing a physician earlier rather than later, like having new tires put on your car before you have a blowout. In the lexicon of cancer researchers, prevention means early examinations, pap smears, and diagnostic X-rays. It does *not* mean eliminating carcinogens in the air and in food products.[80] And more emphatically, it does not mean the dissemination of hard information to the public about what is killing them. By even conservative estimates, 80 to 85 percent of cancers are "extrinsic"—they originate outside the body.[81] Yet cancer research hones curative techniques—radical surgery, radiation, and drugs. In 1972, the National Cancer Institute spent $75 million to test chemicals for cancer treatment. Only four were approved for use on humans, at a cost of slightly less than $20 million per agent.[82] But drugs seem to be the game plan for the future. Dr. Gordon Zubrod, Director of the National Cancer Institute's Division of Cancer Treatment, states flatly, "Surgery and radiation have reached a dead end."[83] So drugs will be the weapons of the future, used in combination with surgery and radiation therapy. Detroit and Winston-Salem should be happy.

Modern medical care focuses on disease and ignores health. The "cure" of symptoms is the objective of treatment. Prevention and public health are lean step-children, in part because medicine has chosen cures over prevention, but also because the public refuses to force medicine to reassess its choice. The pattern of medical practice is mirrored in medical research. The objective of most research is identification of treatments and cures, not, except in a limited way, prevention. In this sense the research world matches the world of practice. Neither is interested in promoting health. Both seek only to eliminate disease. But there is a great difference. Based on current trends, by the year 2000, 1.2 million new cases of cancer will be detected each year in the United States, and about half a million people will die of cancer annually. Most of these 1.7 million people are alive today, since cancer is largely a disease of old age. And most are now eating, inhaling, and drinking the agents that will ultimately kill them. It should be comforting to them to know that in the year 2000 they will have a chance to be "cured" with new and refined tools, sophisticated radiation equipment, and fresh and powerful drugs. And while they are either being "cured," or are dying, their children and their children's children will be eating, inhaling, and drinking the same agents that killed their parents.

4

Medicine: A.D. 2000

For which of you, intending to build a tower, sitteth not down first, and counteth the cost, whether he have sufficient to finish it?

Luke 14:28

Some institutions have trouble learning. Through interaction with their environment, organisms and, homologously, institutions are buffeted by feedback. But some absorb the information more effectively than others. The dinosaur did not absorb information very effectively. The medical care system is the dinosaur of institutions. The resistance of the medical care system to change, and the intransigence of its keepers, is legendary. But medicine must change, because the society in which it is embedded is changing.

"Futurology" is not a science; it is largely in the realm of art. Some relatively concrete methodologies lend some precision to projections about the future, but their application does not inevitably result in any greater accuracy than can be achieved with less formal approaches. The noted futurologist Herman Kahn, in his major book, *The Year 2000: A Framework for Speculation on the Next Thirty-Three Years,* published in 1967, failed even to mention the possibility of "pollution."[1]

Moreover, all futurologists have biases about the future. This alone makes it difficult to conceive of a pure methodol-

ogy of futurology. Charles Hampden-Turner, writing in
Radical Man, makes the point aptly:

> the projection of present trends into the future represents a
> vote of temporary approval for such trends. Yet the trends
> themselves are the consequences of thousands of individual
> human decisions . . . the decision not to change directions [is] a
> decision. By concentrating upon the technical and material
> aspects of these trends, the impression is fostered that things
> "are" like stars and planets around us, so that the "realistic"
> men must humbly subordinate their minds to these physical
> "facts." . . .
>
> But these projections of existing trends are quite *unlike* the
> physical universe of dead objects. They are *cultural, political*
> and *social* choices. Men have the capacity to rebel against any
> trend at any time in any place by deciding to stop it or alter its
> direction, or persuade others to do so. . . . the shared expecta-
> tion that the trend whose direction you oppose will not be
> continued in the future may be politically essential to any
> success in halting or redirecting it.
>
> The obverse is also true. The acceptance of a trend which is
> implicit in projecting into the future, the gathering together of
> technical statistics, scholarly opinion, and humanistic concerns
> about what this trend will mean by the year 2000, had the
> *inevitable effect of strengthening that trend and making it more certain
> to occur.*[2]

As I have said, our approach to health will necessarily
change because our views about health will change—there
are trends and forces at work that will alter our thinking
about health. What follows is a sample of these trends.

YOUNG AND OLD: CHANGES IN
AGE COMPOSITION

Approximately 10 percent of the United States population,
or about 20 million persons, are age 65 or older. Two factors
directly affect the proportion of the aged in the population,
the birth rate and the aging process.

In 1960, the birth rate was 23.7 per 1000 people; in 1970, the rate descended to 18.2.[3] Since then the data show an even greater decline—the number of children per family declined from 3.5 in 1960 to 2.136 in March 1972.[4] Demographers attribute these declines in part to disincentives. The desire to have a lot of children is not great in a society where most children survive to maturity. The impact of information about population pressures provided by the government, or by activist movements such as Zero Population Growth and the Commission on Population Growth and the American Future may also be appreciable.[5] On the assumption that children born in this century will enjoy a favorable prognosis for survival, and that population stabilization programs will flourish, the birth rate will probably continue to drop or will at least plateau. Hence, by the year 2000 and in the absence of other major demographic changes, there will be relatively more older persons than now.[6]

A second factor affecting the proportion of elders in the population is the aging process. Predictions about advances in medical science are patently risky, but Alexander Comfort, a physician and expert on the aging process, has stated that "there is a real possibility of a breakthrough affecting human vigor at high ages, or the human life span, or both."[7] Dr. Comfort elaborates on these points in his book, *The Process of Aging.*[8] He argues that any single palliative such as a cure for atherosclerosis, a principal cause of strokes and heart attacks, would result in some persons growing older, but that the effect on longevity would not be dramatic. But, while a radical lengthening of the life span is unlikely in the absence of a profound retardation of the aging process, a mode age in the high 70s or low 80s might occur. Assuming no dramatic life-prolonging technologies, then, the year 2000 may witness a much older population—in absolute numbers, around 35 million, and in percentages, perhaps 12 to 15 percent of the population.[9]

This will affect medical care in three ways. First, there are

few geriatric specialists, although there are hordes of pediatricians. There is a geriatric medicine, but specialization in
geriatrics is not common. Currently 17,941 pediatricians
practice in the United States. Based on an AMA survey, only
117 physicians of the 40 percent of the physicians who
responded to the survey classify themselves as geria-
tricians.[10] This means that the ratios are one doctor for
every 4300 persons under 19,[11] and roughly one for every
67,000 over 65 (based on a population of 20 million over 65
and extrapolating the survey response to a final figure of
300 geriatric practitioners). The ratios will decrease even
further by the year 2000 unless more specialists are trained
to deal with the health problems of the aged.

Second, degenerative diseases of old age, atherosclerosis,
heart disease, some cancers, and miscellaneous chronic disabling conditions like arthritis and rheumatism are among
the diseases upon which medicine has the least impact.[12]
Elders do incur infectious diseases that can be successfully
treated, and their brittle bones can be set if they break, but
many diseases from which they suffer can only be tempered,
and their pain can only be modulated. Medicine has contributed to the preservation of life, but medicine can only
maintain persons who sustain most illnesses associated with
aging.

Third, medical care resources are disproportionately allocated to those over 65. In fiscal 1970, the average annual
medical bill for an aged person was $791, compared to $123
for a child and $296 for those between 19 and 65. The aged
currently constitute roughly 10 percent of the population,
but roughly 27 percent of medical care expenditures were
made by and on their behalf. Public funds, principally Medicare expenditures, accounted for about 60 percent.[13]

What do these data mean? The public outlay of dollars for
medical care for those over 65 rose rapidly after 1966, the
year Medicare was enacted. Since then, adjusting for population and price increases, the annual increase in personal

health care expenditures for the aged has averaged 9.2 percent. If this increase persists until the year 2000 and assuming neither a dramatic increase in life span nor price increase (and even assuming that only 10 percent of the total population will be 65 and over in the year 2000), the $15.7 billion now spent for medical care for the aged will leap to $220.1 billion. And assuming a climb from 10 percent to 15 percent of those over 65, with no change in life span and no inflation, expenditures will reach $336.9 billion. Attaching an inflation rate of 6.2 percent per year, or roughly the rate of inflation from 1966 to 1970, a bill for medical care services for the aged will be delivered in the year 2000 for $2,047,000,000,000, or more than two trillion dollars.[14]

Of course, the figures exaggerate the increases because they are based on inherently unstable linear projections. But in a rough sense the figures do show that medical care for the aged is very costly, and will become much more costly if the public tolerates it. The result is unhappy in any event, since the care that now is provided to the aged is palliative at best. And this will be the case in the year 2000 unless we recognize that the aged need care, but not necessarily medical care.

The problem is cast into sharp relief when the nursing home issue is added. Thousands of aged persons are currently housed in nursing homes.[15] Others are warehoused in mental health institutions because of the lack of nursing home beds or other places for the poor and elderly. Historically the nursing home has been thought of largely as shelter. A more contemporary view is that the nursing home should be a less elaborate hospital. Many elders need medical care, but since it is largely palliative, few of them achieve self-sufficiency. They are kept on the pap of the institution where they have been housed. Other countries, such as Denmark and Sweden, less influenced by the medical model and more by a mix of realism and compassion, have been successful in springing the elderly from these institutional traps. As long as they are stacked like so much wood into institutions, the aged will steadily become a more deeply dependent class and a costly one at that. Either medicine must develop the means to cure the diseases of old age, at a price that will become exorbitant for genteel bedside manners and prescriptions for bedsores, or society must rethink how it will care for the aged.

All the blame cannot be placed on medicine. A coherent policy for the aged has not been formulated in this country. As a result, the medical care system has become the caretaker for countless older persons whom society chooses to ignore. Both nursing homes and mental health institutions count among their patients many who could be better (and probably more inexpensively) placed elsewhere. An elder who is not fully capable of self-care should not be assigned to a treatment center designed for the helpless. Medical care and housing for the aged are not disparate needs but rather points along a continuum of need—there are those who are wholly competent and those who are patently incompetent. But since medicine only rarely heals and often coarsely maintains the elderly—hardware and clinical detachment are poor substitutes for love and care—it should not be asked to solve all of their problems.

SHIFTS IN DISEASE PATTERNS

The environmental factors that induce stress are growing in number. Alvin Toffler in *Future Shock*[16] and Donald Schoen in *Beyond the Stable State*[17] discuss some of these factors. Nearly exponential increases in the amount and volume of noise, automobile traffic, and related phenomena are among the major contributors.

Research on stress, principally by Hans Selye, has unveiled a relatively common bodily response to stressful conditions. Selye refers to it as the "General Adaptation Syndrome."

The term "adaptation" is used because the body reacts by trying to adapt to or resist the threat.[18]

Linkages between stress and specific diseases have not been conclusively established in many cases. However, disease, which many consider related to stress, is on the march. René Dubos puts it this way:

> Cancer, heart disease, and disorders of the cerebral system are commonly referred to as diseases of civilization. Strictly speaking, the designation is incorrect, since these diseases occur also among the primitive peoples. Such chronic and degenerative conditions are so much more frequent among prosperous peoples than among primitive or economically deprived groups that it is justifiable to speak of "diseases of civilization." The very use of that phrase is tacit acknowledgement that our ways of life may have nefarious effects and that affluence, like poverty, can constitute a cause of disease.[19]

The data are supportive. Figure 7 illustrates the nature of mortality today as distinguished from the turn of the century. From 1900 to 1967, as a percentage of all deaths, vascular lesions affecting the central nervous system rose from 6.2 percent to 10.9 percent, and diseases of the heart from 8.0 percent to 39.0 percent (see Figure 7). These "diseases of civilization," to use Dubos's phrase, do not just rise with the population but increase in incidence, controlling for population. For example, the increase in the rate per 100,000 population for heart disease jumped from 137 in 1900 to 364.5 in 1967, although it is recently trailing off (see Figure 7).

The causation is often unknown, but socioenvironmental stresses can influence the onset of disease. These factors are unlikely to disappear. There is no reason to assume that the conditions that cause stress will abate in the next 30 years. On the contrary, society in the year 2000 will probably be more ennervating, swifter in pace, noisier, and more bellicose than it is now. Stress is related to the pace of change,

FIGURE 7   THE 10 LEADING CAUSES OF U.S. DEATHS, 1900
AND 1968

Rank Order and	Cause of Death	Death Rate per 100,000 Population	Percentage of Deaths
1900			
Deaths from all causes		1719	100.0
1.	Major cardiovascular-renal diseases	345.2	20.0
2.	Influenza and pneumonia	202.2	11.8
3.	Tuberculosis, all forms	194.4	11.3
4.	Gastritis, duodenitis, enteritis and and colitis (diarrhea)	142.7	8.3
5.	Accidents	72.3	4.2
6.	Cancer	64.0	3.7
7.	Diphtheria	40.3	2.3
8.	Typhoid and Paratyphoid fever	31.3	1.8
9.	Measles	13.3	.8
10.	Cirrhosis of the liver	12.5	.7
1968			
Deaths from all causes		970	100.0
1.	Diseases of the heart	372.6	38.4
2.	Cancer	159.4	16.4
3.	Cerebrovascular diseases	105.8	10.9
4.	Accidents	57.5	5.9
5.	Influenza and pneumonia	36.8	3.8
6.	Certain diseases of early infancy	21.9	2.3
7.	Diabetes mellitus	19.2	2.0
8.	Arteriosclerosis	16.8	1.7
9.	Bronchitis, emphysema, and asthma	16.6	1.7
10.	Cirrhosis of the liver	14.6	1.5

Source. U.S. Department of Commerce, Bureau of the Census, *Historical Statistics of the U.S., Colonial Times to 1957* (Washington, D.C.: U.S. Government Printing Office, 1960), p. 26, and *Statistical Abstract of the U.S.: 1972,* 93d ed. (Washington, D.C.: U.S. Government Printing Office, 1972), p. 60.

and despite accumulated evidence of man's inherent adaptability, there may be a ceiling to adaptation. To quote Dubos again:

the rate of change is so rapid that there may not be time for the orderly and successful operation of these conscious and unconscious adaptive processes. For the first time in the history of mankind, the biological and social experience of the father is almost useless to the son.[20]

There is other supporting evidence. One of the diseases generally thought to be related to stress is hypertension, or high blood pressure. Cassel and Leighton write:

> Studies on blood pressure, for example, conducted in many countries across the world, including Brazil, Guatemala, South Africa, Easter Islands, Fiji and the Gilbert Islands, and the New Hebrides have shown that populations living in small cohesive societies "insulated" from the changes that are occurring in the Western industrializing countries tend to have low blood pressures which do not differ in the young and the aged. In a number of these studies, groups who have left these societies and had contact with Western culture were also examined and found to have higher levels of blood pressure and to exhibit the familiar relationship between age and blood pressure found in studies of Western populations.[21]

Variations in hypertensivity also arise within cultures and seem in part due to occupational and residential mobility. Job loss appears to be highly related.[22] Cassel and Leighton add:

> Studies in the U.S. have demonstrated that occupationally and residentially mobile people have higher prevalence rates of coronary heart disease than have stable populations, and that stable rural residents have increasing mortality rates from coronary heart disease as the county in which they live becomes more urbanized.[23]

Hypertension presents two special problems to medicine. First, there are many more cases of hypertension than those under treatment. It is a difficult disorder to detect because most people who have it do not know it—there are no classic symptoms. Recent screenings, many sponsored by local Heart Associations, revealed anywhere from 12.5 to 30 percent of those screened to be hypertensive. The second problem arises from the treatment. For those few who are under treatment, the cure is often worse than the disease. Hypertension is generally treated with a battery of medications, most of which have side effects ranging from the mildly unpleasant to the downright noxious. But one fact remains: on the average the hypertensive lives 17 years less than those without the condition.[24]

Hypertension is only one stress-related disease. Research on the incidence of disease among Navy and Marine personnel is illustrative.[25] Based on a longitudinal examination of the health records of 15 men, illnesses clustered immediately after "life-changes." The "life-changes" most highly related to the onset of illness were loss of a spouse, divorce, imprisonment, and loss of a family member. Also, a study reported in 1972 by Holmes and Masuda linked illness with many of the same factors identified in the study of Navy and Marine personnel.[26]

Two other studies focused on some unique stress conditions. In the first, Kasl and Cobb sought to link parental status anxiety with disease in their children. Their findings partially supported their hypothesis that "status stress" affected the health of their offspring. Women with arthritis were more likely to come from families with "high-status-stress." But no relationship was found between stress levels and arthritis in men and ulcers for both men and women. The children of both sexes from families with "high-status-stress," however, possessed negative "attitudes" about health. They thought they were in poor health, were frequently depressed, and manifested more physical symptoms of anxiety and low energy.[27]

The second study suggests that if stress is enough to get one into the hospital, things might get worse. Skipper and

Leonard found, independent of illness, that children hospitalized for tonsillectomy and their mothers often experienced heightened stress, including elevated temperature, pulse, and blood pressure levels, disturbed sleep, and protracted periods of recovery after treatment. The hospital setting for some then might complicate rather than enhance recuperation.[28]

There are cost implications as well. Current therapies for many of these diseases—cobalt therapy, heart surgery, hyperbaric chambers for certain surgical procedures—are extremely expensive. Biomedical research is itself also very costly. In 1972, National Institute of Health expenditures for heart and lung research alone totaled $232,969,000. In 1974, biomedical research for cancer alone reached $589 million, out of a total of more than $1.5 billion for all federally supported biomedical research.[29]

The point is that the diseases that afflict a given culture vary with the social and physical conditions that characterize the culture. Contemporary life, because it is so stressful, can induce certain kinds of disease—in some cases diseases related directly to stress, like hypertension. In yet other cases, contemporary life increases the incidence of diseases such as gastric disorders, heart failure, and perhaps some cancers. But there are some qualifying factors. First, the argument that stress can induce, or at least heighten, susceptibility to disease only indirectly supports the idea that stress-related diseases are more prevalent today because of higher levels of stress. There are persuasive arguments that stress is greater because life is more grinding and more ennervating than in the past. But the studies discussed in this section traced the impact on health of factors such as divorce, loss of a spouse, and so on, which are not unique to contemporary life. Thus, although arguments about the rise in prevalence of stress-related disease are probably sound, the research support is sketchy.

A second qualifying note might be contained in this question, what can be done about stress? Life is complex and fast, and nothing can be done about it. This is only partially true. It will be difficult to alter the conditions of life that create stress, but not impossible. And to do so might have a real payoff. Medicine cannot cure the diseases associated with stress, and the prognosis for miracle cures is not good. If this is the case, why not assault the conditions that cause stress? To do so cannot be that much more difficult than finding cures. I return to this issue.

Finally, examination of epidemiological data reveals an intriguing fact. Not only have increases in life span been slowing, recent evidence shows a plateau in the life expectancy of white males over 55 in the United States since about the mid-fifties, and stabilization in the rate for the rest of the population.[30] Medicine may no longer extend longevity and may, given the damage resulting from the impact of other factors, be losing the battle to prolong life. Our life spans may soon begin to contract.

SELF-INFLICTED MORBIDITY AND MORTALITY

The number of injuries from accidents, controlling for population, has remained roughly stable over the last 20 years, although rate increases have been experienced in motor vehicle use (see Figure 8). But even though accidents are not increasing faster than population growth, the toll is staggering. More than 120,000 people die in accidents each year. Traffic accidents alone account for nearly one-half of these deaths. An additional 50 million persons are injured, 5 million in auto accidents. These injuries combine to consume 22 million hospital bed days per year.[31] The Insurance Information Institute estimates that if current automotive use patterns persist, 86,000 persons will die in accidents in 1980, and 6,460,000 will be injured. By extrapolation, again based on current motor vehicle use, there will be 200,000 deaths annually from automotive use alone by the year 2000.[32] Of course, any major decrease in automobile use or significant improvement in auto safety in the next 30 years would render these projections unreliable.

The incidence of injury is linked with age. The young are disproportionately the victims in fatal traffic accidents, and accidental injuries and deaths bear more heavily on the aged, particularly because of protracted recuperation. The confluence of increasing accident rates and increases in the number of older persons will result in greater mortality and morbidity among the aged.[33]

Between 1940 and 1968, the annual consumption of alcohol rose from 1.48 gallons per capita to 2.37 gallons per capita. Beer consumption rose from 18.22 gallons to 25.88 gallons per capita for the same period.[34] The National Institute of Alcohol Abuse and Alcoholism points out that 68 percent of United States citizens drink, and about 9 million Americans are either alcoholics or nearly so. The Institute refers to alcoholism as the nation's "largest untreated treatable disease."[35]

Similarly, addictive drug use has steadily increased in recent years. The number of reported addicts in 1971 was 23,881, as against the average for the period 1953 to 1971 of 8587.[36] Finally, evidence of the link between smoking and lung cancer has not significantly dampened smoking—all that has happened is a decrease in the rate of increase. And according to recent data, it may not make too much difference whether a person smokes, since a nonsmoker exposed to cigarette smoke may suffer some of the same consequences.[37]

In the next three decades the costs of medical care will steadily rise. Many more practitioners will be trained,[38] and the use of high technology procedures will increase. During this same period, deaths from auto accidents could rise from 56,000 per year to about 200,000, and the consumption of distilled spirits spurt from roughly 2.4 gallons to 3.8 gallons

FIGURE 8 DEATHS AND DEATH RATES FROM ACCIDENTS, 1950 TO 1968[a]

Type of Accident	Deaths					Rate[b]				
	1950	1955	1960	1965	1968	1950	1955	1960	1965	1968
All accidents	91,249	93,443	93,806	108,004	114,864	60.6	56.9	52.3	55.7	57.5
Railway accidents	2,126	1,344	1,023	962	849	1.4	0.8	0.6	0.5	0.4
Motor vehicle accidents	34,763	38,426	38,137	49,163	54,862	23.1	23.4	21.3	25.4	27.5
Traffic	33,863	37,437	37,142	48,050	53,801	22.5	22.8	20.7	24.8	26.9
Nontraffic	900	989	995	1,113	1,061	0.6	0.6	0.6	0.6	0.5
Other road vehicle accidents	533	330	243	319	264	0.4	0.2	0.1	0.2	0.1
Water transport accidents	1,502	1,452	1,478	1,493	1,625	1.0	0.9	0.8	0.8	0.8
Aircraft accidents	1,436	1,446	1,475	1,529	1,904	1.0	0.9	0.8	0.8	1.0
Accidental poisoning by										
Solid and liquid substances	1,584	1,431	1,679	2,110	2,583	1.1	0.9	0.9	1.1	1.3
Gases and vapors	1,769	1,163	1,253	1,526	1,526	1.2	0.7	0.7	0.8	0.8
Accidental falls	20,783	20,192	19,023	19,984	18,651	13.8	12.3	10.6	10.3	9.3
From one level to another	7,117	6,811	6,019	5,802	5,034	4.7	4.1	3.4	3.0	2.5
On the same level	4,569	4,275	3,689	5,738	958	3.0	2.6	2.1	3.0	0.5
Unspecified	9,097	9,106	9,315	8,444	12,659	6.0	5.5	5.2	4.4	6.3
Blow from falling object	1,613	1,332	1,404	1,493	1,393	1.1	0.8	0.8	0.8	0.7

Accidents caused by									
Machinery	1,771	2,019	1,951	2,054	(NA)	1.2	1.2	1.1	1.1	(NA)
Electric current	955	1,075	989	1,071	1,048	0.6	0.7	0.6	0.6	0.5
Fire and explosion, etc	6,405	6,352	7,645	7,347	7,977	4.3	3.9	4.3	3.8	4.0
Hot substances, etc	842	742	402	420	278	0.6	0.5	0.2	0.2	0.1
Firearms	2,174	2,120	2,334	2,344	2,394	1.4	1.3	1.3	1.2	1.2
Inhalation and ingestion of objects	1,350	1,608	2,397	1,836	3,100	0.9	1.0	1.3	0.9	1.6
Accidental drowning	4,785	5,046	5,232	5,485	5,950	3.2	3.1	2.9	2.8	3.0
Excessive heat and insolation	137	615	168	106	231	0.1	0.4	0.1	0.1	0.1
Complications due to medical procedures	589	776	1,115	1,494	2,023	0.4	0.5	0.6	0.8	1.0
All other accidents	6,132	5,974	5,858	7,268	8,206	4.1	3.6	3.3	3.7	4.1

Source. U.S. Department of Commerce, Bureau of the Census, *Statistical Abstract of the United States, 1972,* 93d ed. (Washington, D.C.: U.S. Government Printing Office, 1972), p. 61.

[a] Prior to 1960, excludes Alaska and Hawaii. NA = not available.

[b] Per 100,000 resident population. For 1950 and 1960, based on population enumerated as of April 1; for other years, based on population estimated as of July 1.

per capita.[39] Aside from participating in some automobile
accidents and consuming their share of the alcohol, physicians will do little to prevent this loss.

Accidents. Accidents present two interrelated medical care
problems. The first is the patent inadequacy of emergency
care services. According to the U.S. Public Health Service
and the National Safety Council, accidental trauma killed
114,000 persons and permanently impaired 500,000 more in
1971 alone.[40] Trauma is initially handled by the emergency
care subsystem of the medical care system. Arthur Freese in
the *Saturday Review* assessed the adequacy of emergency
services.[41] A publication of the National Research Council of
the National Academy of Sciences, referred to by Freese,
describes trauma as "the neglected epidemic of modern society." In Chicago, according to a study conducted by the
Chicago Hospital Council, an average of 804 "emergency"
cases are transported to hospitals per week in police
"squadrols"—paddy wagons that also carry drunks and in-
mates. Oxygen is not available to the 35 cardiac cases per
week, nor to the 51 cases of seizures/convulsions, nor to the
21 persons who are unconscious when picked up. In addition, the 179 limb injuries cannot be splinted, nor can the
200 lacerations be treated.[42]

The emergency care problem does not stem from inadequacy of the medical care provided once the victim reaches
the hospital (although the emergency room is the abattoir of
medicine—only one out of six hospitals in the United States
staff emergency facilities with physicians on a 24-hour basis),
but rather from the services rendered by the freight haulers
who pick up the body and transport it to the hospital. For
example, in a study of 159 highway fatalities in Michigan,
discussed by Freese, the investigators concluded that 37
might have survived if prompt and effective treatment had
been rendered at the scene of the accident.[43] Unless physi-

cians attend all ambulance calls, which is unlikely, more lives might be saved by improving emergency treatment of trauma than by spending more money on hospitals.

But perhaps physicians should attend all ambulance calls. The treatment of acutely ill or injured people is one of the things medicine does well. Most studies of emergency care conclude that lives could be saved if the injured could be brought to the hospital sooner.

The emergency care problem exemplifies the "boundary conditions" of medicine. To test medicine by the test of effectiveness is likely to result in a contraction of its "boundaries"—limiting medicine to what works. But medicine might also expand its boundaries. Emergency care is a leading candidate. One reason so much damage is done in emergency situations is that, unlike all other medical care settings, there is no single locus of responsibility. Sometimes the police are involved, sometimes the sheriff, and sometimes bystanders. Sometimes a police ambulance is deployed, but most of the time a private outfit performs the run. But in all cases, medicine, like the expectant father, sits and waits for the patient to be delivered. In the meantime other agencies stumble over each other with the life of the victim in the balance. This is as tragic as it is foolish. Medicine can save and heal severely injured patients and it could do so by taking charge of emergency care.

The second and larger problem is not necessarily amenable to medicine. We have not insisted that medical care orient itself to prevention. In Chapter 2, some of the cost-benefit findings relating to medical services were discussed. As noted there, crude cost-benefit analyses have been constructed comparing the impact of certain disease control programs. The prevention programs that were analyzed involved simple measures such as use of seat belts and defensive driving techniques. And a high benefit-to-cost ratio was calculated. To further illustrate, Figure 9 is drawn from a study by the Joint Economic Committee of the U.S.

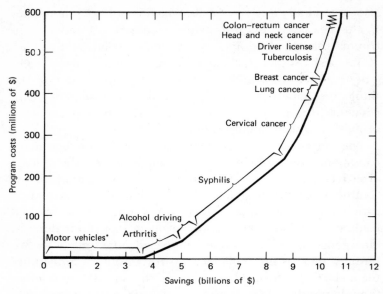

FIGURE 9   DOLLAR SAVING IN CANCER PROGRAMS COMPARED
TO OTHER TREATMENT PROGRAMS

Source.   The Analysis and Evaluation of Public Expenditures: The PPB System
(U.S. Congress, Joint Economics Committee, Subcommittee on Economy in
Government, 1969).

Note.   The cost for motor vehicles includes that of programs on use of seat
belts, defensive driving, and reduction in pedestrian injuries.

Congress. As the figure demonstrates, there are some clear
trade offs in the costs and benefits of various programs. For
example, if the estimates by the committee are accurate, is
the savings of $3 billion through programs of driver educa-
tion and safety for a cost of a few million dollars a better
social investment than a potential saving of $8.5 billion
through treatment of cervical cancer at a cost of $300 to 400
million? In the first case the cost-benefit ratio is roughly
1:1,000 (assuming a program cost of $3 million); in the
second it is 1:25. Even though it costs far less to undertake
the former program than the latter, I would not want to
make the judgment to save a driver or a person afflicted

with cervical cancer. But medicine makes that decision every day by dragooning the resources to treat the latter that could be spent for the former.

Chemicals. One of every seven patients has a drinking problem, according to the Alcohol and Drug Dependence Clinic in Memphis, Tennessee.[44] Dr. David H. Knott, medical director of the clinic, reproaches his fellow practitioners this way: "We've gotten too hung up diagnosing alcohol dependency in terms of how much an individual drinks, how often he drinks, how many years he's been drinking. . . . [I]nstead we should be more concerned with the more subtle effects that alcohol has on an individual's health and ability to function." The opportunity for medicine to do more may be dawning.[45] Today, with a few exceptions, the alcoholic in our society is classified as a criminal and treated by "drying out." But alcoholism is being steadily decriminalized and alcoholics transferred to the medical care system. And although we do not know as much as we should about the causes and cures of alcoholism, there are a few therapies that appear to work. But effective treatment is seldom afforded. Society has refused to pay enough for it, and an insufficient number of physicians have been trained to provide it.

Then there are other drugs. Alcohol is probably the most dangerous; it incapacitates more people than other chemicals. But while figures are hard to get, undoubtedly heroin, other opium derivatives, "downers," and "uppers" also account for a substantial amount of morbidity and some deaths as well. The well-publicized deaths of public figures including Marilyn Monroe, Jimi Hendrix, and Janis Joplin are examples.

The real challenge lies in the design of programs to deal with drug and alcohol use and dependency. To some, like Andrew Weil, society must first recognize the "positive" aspects of drug use, while not necessarily fostering its wider use.[46] But to many others, "treatment" and deterrence are the goals, despite the bleakness of the record.

Whatever the result of the debate, two things are reasonably clear. Alcohol and drug use are not wholly medical problems. Many of the causes of chemical dependency escape medicine's grasp as well as its tools. Although physicians can help, chemical dependency is a "boundary condition." But even if medicine expanded its boundaries to embrace the millions who are now in bondage to chemicals, it would fail.

Second, there is the expense. Approximately 120,000 drug users are currently under treatment. If they all were hospitalized, the cost of treatment alone would exceed $4 billion per year. In contrast, the treatment of addicts through methadone maintenance would cost about $160 million.[47] Even if medical treatment worked as well as methadone maintenance, and we do not know whether it would, the cost would be roughly 30 times as great. It is one example, among many, where the medical solution to a problem is far more costly than other solutions.

The issue of whether the medical model will be deployed to deal with problems of deviance, like drug abuse, is an important issue, particularly because there is little evidence that it will work. But the more important issue is how to slow down the rate of chemical use. The rates of consumption for most drugs, including alcohol, are steadily increasing. In the wake of those increases come increased health hazards. And we encourage the disease—more than $250 million is spent per year to advertise liquor, as per capita alcohol consumption inexorably grows. Heroin addiction is almost epidemic in some urban areas. And even greater increases are reported in the use of both barbiturates ("downers") and amphetamines ("uppers"). The Consumers Union, in *Licit and Illicit Drugs,* reports staggering increases.[48] Even aspirin use has reached huge proportions. More than 20,000 tons of aspirin are consumed annually in the United States—225 tablets per person per year.[49]

And beyond those chemicals we willingly and knowingly consume, there are a host of others secreted in foodstuffs and other consumables which slowly chip away at our health. Figure 10 contains estimates of the impact chemicals have on health and life. Using the maximum figures, more than 50 percent of all deaths in 1967 were linked to chemicals. The data vividly demonstrate that a solution to chemical use and abuse might yield enormous benefits. This then is why the real question is not what "model," criminal, mental or medical, is used to "treat" those who are chronically addicted, but rather what can be done about the causes of chemical abuse.

THE ENVIRONMENT AND ITS ENEMIES

The Club of Rome, a group of academicians, statesmen, philanthropists, and concerned nonspecialists, issued its first report in 1972 as a part of its continuing examination of the "predicament of mankind." The major conclusion in its report, *The Limits to Growth*,[50] is that "if the present growth trends in world population, industrialization, pollution, food production and resource depletion continue unchanged, the limits to growth . . . will be reached some time within the next 100 years."[51]

Assuming the Club of Rome is wrong, or at least slightly off target, most of us will survive the impending ecological catastrophe. But we will suffer the ravages of environmental degradation nevertheless, as will our heirs. There is a substantial amount of theory on this subject which is systematically being supported by research. Despite the research, the growth issue remains highly controversial.[52] But an unmistakable fact is that our environment is being plundered and, new technology notwithstanding, conditions will worsen in the next few decades.

FIGURE 10 NUMBERS AND PERCENTAGES OF DEATHS IN 1967 LINKED TO VARIOUS CHEMICAL FACTORS[a]

Numbers of Deaths Linked to Factor in 1967	Percentage of All Deaths in 1967 Linked to Factor	Factor	Adjusted Percentages of Death Allowing for Age at which Death Occurs	
			Adjustment A	Adjustment B
300,000	17	Cigarette smoking	13	8
56,000	3	Alcohol abuse[b]	6	9
0 to 400,000	0 to 20	Dietary composition	0 to 13	0 to 8
60,000 to 150,000	3 to 8	Unknown factors which act as initiators and promoters of cancer	3 to 7	2 to 5
75,000	4	Adverse reactions to medication	1.4	1.2
10,000	0.6	Narcotic and addictive drugs	1.2	1.2
9,000	0.5	Community air pollution	0.3	0.1
9,000	0.5	Airborne particles (occupational)	0.3	0.1
4,600	0.25	Suicides involving chemicals	0.5	0.7
2,800	0.15	Coffee drinking (bladder cancer)	0.1	0.03
2,200	0.01	Accidents with chemicals	0.25	0.35
150	0.01	Oral contraceptives	0.02	0.04

Source. Chemicals and Health, Report of the Panel on Chemicals and Health of the President's Science Advisory Committee, September 1973 (Washington, D.C., U.S. Government Printing Office, 1973), p. 35.

[a] 100% = total deaths from all causes = 1,850,000.

[b] Includes accidental deaths in which alcohol was a contributor as well as diseases primarily linked to alcohol.

Although nearly all experts acknowledge the ecological price exacted by development, most of the arguments can be plotted along two dimensions. Along the first, experts range themselves on the question of the degree of pollution, now and in the future. The polar positions are occupied, respectively, by those who believe the earth's resources to be nearly inexhaustible and those who forecast inescapable disaster. The Club of Rome meets near the latter pole.

A second dimension concerns whether current trends can be reversed by the application of new technology to undo what has been done. Neo-Luddites occupy one pole, while apologists for industry stand at the other. To quote former President Nixon on the subject, the solution to the environmental crisis is to rely on "the same reservoir of inventive genius that created . . . problems in the first place." But Barry Commoner, in *The Closing Circle,* makes the case that new technology cannot be harnessed to cure what old technology has put asunder.[53] Although Commoner recognizes that some technological hardware might be used to curb some pollution, he isolates fault in the very heart of the science which nourishes technology:

> There is, indeed, a specific fault in our system of science, and in the resultant understanding of the natural world which, I believe, helps to explain the ecological failure of technology. This fault is reductionism, the view that effective understanding of a complex system can be achieved by investigating the properties of its isolated parts. The reductionist methodology, which is so characteristic of much of modern research, is not an effective means of analyzing the vast natural systems that are threatened by degradation.[54]

The remedy seems to lie both in the stabilization of growth itself, with selected reductions and transformations of specific processes, practices, and preferences, and in the application of a purified, holistic technology. However, there is little likelihood that the radical changes in life style that would be necessary to achieve stable growth will occur in the next 30 years. Moreover, even assuming the brake is vigorously applied in the United States, growth will continue unchecked elsewhere in the world. This, in simple form, is Garrett Hardin's "tragedy of the commons."[55] Commoner and Hardin are not alone in this view. The Club of Rome and others have reached the same conclusion.

The Environment and Health.   The causes of cancer surround us. It is easier to treat a cut, set a bone, or remove a diseased organ than to eliminate carcinogens in the air we breathe. We can try to do both but there are costs and trade offs, and today we stress treatment of the sick and neglect the cure of conditions that induce sickness. One of the simplest ways to demonstrate the point is to examine the differences in mortality for people with different habits. Figure 11 speaks for

FIGURE 11   DAYS LIFE EXPECTANCY LOST PER 65 YEARS EXPOSURE

Fallout from all atomic weapons tests to date	−1.2 days
Cosmic rays, sea level	−22 days
Wearing luminous dial watch	−26 days
Cosmic rays, 5000 feet	−33 days
Living over sedimentary rock	−50 days
Medical and dental X-rays	−64 days and more
Living over granitic rock	−94 days
Living in brick or concrete homes	−100–200 days
Use of antibiotics, when necessary	+730 days
25% overweight	−1300 days
Living in the city (in contrast to rural living)	−1800 days
Sedentary, in contrast to an active life	−about 1800 days
Smoking, one pack per day	−3300 days
Diabetes, insulin controlled	−3600 days
Women, in contrast to men, will gain	1100 days
Married people will live longer than single people by	1800 days

Source.   Data from the American Heart Association and the Department of Health, Education, and Welfare.

itself; it illustrates what Robert Rushmer, a physician now at the University of Washington Bio-Engineering Laboratory, calls "sui-sickness," disability and even death resulting from suicidal impulses.

Environmental factors—polluted air and water, noise, stress—are the most important determinants of ill health. If this is so, and if environmental conditions linked to health worsen over the next 30 years, the future promises more business for physicians but poorer health for everyone. Pollutants induce a wide range of biological effects in man that are generically and collectively termed "toxicity." Acute or chronic toxicity may be manifested in fetal, neonatal, perinatal, childhood, or adult life; the effects range from impairment of functioning to death. Cancer, birth defects, and mutations, among other afflictions, are caused by environmental pollutants. And tragically, sustained exposure to new synthetic chemicals and their by-products in our air, water, and soil may result both in intensification of known diseases and the discovery of still others.[56]

But there are gaps in our information—more is known about certain pollutants than others. Nevertheless, as a general proposition, environmental pollution creates three health hazards. The first is cancer. While not conclusive, there is growing recognition that the majority of cancers are due to chemical carcinogens in the environment. The pandemic incidence of lung cancer in the United States and England has been unequivocally linked with smoking, although air pollution is a contributing factor. The mastication of betel nuts and tobacco leaves results in the high incidence of oral cancers in Asia (oral cancers represent 35 percent of all cancers in Asia, but only 1 percent in Europe). Samuel Epstein, a bacteriologist and sociologist, adds:

> The high incidence of liver cancer among the Bantu and in Guam is probably due to dietary contamination with aflatoxin, a potent fungal carcinogen, and to eating Cycad plants, con-

taining azoxyglucoside carcinogens, respectively. The high incidence of gastric cancer in Japan, Iceland and Chile has been associated with high dietary intake of fish; suggestions have been made implicating nitrosamines, formed by reactions between secondary amines in fish and nitrite preservations. The high incidence of cancer of the esophagus in Zambians drinking Kachasu spirits may be related to its high nitrosamine contamination. A wide range of occupationally induced cancers is also well recognized. These include bladder cancer in the aniline dye and rubber industry, lung cancer in uranium miners of Colorado and in workers in nitrogen mustard factories in Japan, nasal sinus cancer in wood workers. Pleural and peritoneal mesotheliomas in asbestos workers, and skin cancer in shale oil workers.[57]

A second hazard is mutagenicity, mutations due to chemical interference with the genetic process. Radiation was the first suspect. Since then the list has grown, and while the causal link is not complete, the likelihood of mutations through expanded use of mutagenic agents is clear. Mutations can be either dominant, such as early fetal death or abnormality, retinoblastoma, and sterility, or recessive as in the case of albinism, some anemias, and phenylketonuria. Unfortunately, the impact of recessive mutations is not only deferred but may spread over many generations. Abnormalities may also include heightened susceptibility to leukemia, cancers, and alterations in sex ratios.[58]

The dangers of mutation have been understated despite the evidence already available. Only recently has the role of genetics in disease been adequately recognized. Joshua Lederberg, a geneticist, reflects our current understanding of the relationship between genetics and health this way:

If we give proper weight to the genetic component of many common diseases which have a more complex etiology than the textbook examples of Mendelian defects, we can calculate that at least 25 percent of our health burden is of genetic origin. This figure is a very conservative estimate in view of the genetic component of such griefs as schizophrenia, diabetes, atherosclerosis, mental retardation, early senility and many congenital malformations. In fact, the genetic factor in disease is bound to increase to an even larger proportion, for as we deal with infectious disease and other environmental insults, the genetic legacy of the species will compete only with traumatic accidents as the major factor in health.[59]

The third hazard goes by the intriguing name of "tetralogy," structural abnormalities usually recognizable shortly after birth and causing both disability and death. A slightly broader definition includes abnormalities of prenatal origin. The most notorious example of a tetralogical abnormality was the thalidomide disaster of 1962.

A swelling body of research is focused on these major health hazards. A summary of some of the work shows that there is epidemiologic support for a causal relationship between air pollution and lung cancer. There are marked regional differences in lung cancer mortality related to increased urbanization and to increased levels of organic pollutants in the air.[60] Thus, higher lung cancer rates in urban areas cannot be explained only by factors such as smoking or occupation. In a survey completed in 1958, the lung cancer rate in the United States, standardized for smoking habits and age, was 39 per 100,000 population in rural areas and 52 per 100,000 in cities with populations in excess of 50,000.[61] Similar surveys in England confirmed the significance of the urban factor.[62]

The research on environmental health hazards points to the following:

- Based on estimates made by the National Institute of Environmental Health Sciences in 1970, the health cost to the United States for disease caused by environmental misuse was $35 billion per year, of which $10 billion was spent for treatment of disorders. The remainder represented lost wages and services.

- The link between the inhalation of smoke and lung cancer[63] and emphysema was found as early as 1819.[64] With respect to lung cancer, the Public Health Service reported in 1967 that "for the bulk of the population . . . the importance of cigarette smoking as a cause of broncho-pulmonary disease is much greater than that of atmospheric pollution or occupational exposures." The same publication treats heart disease with this gingerly language: "there is increasing convergence of many types of evidence concerning cigarette smoking and coronary heart disease which strongly suggests that cigarette smoking can cause death from coronary heart disease."[65] Subsequent PHS publications are more forthright in their conclusions. In later reports smoking and air contaminants are linked to chronic bronchitis, emphysema, spontaneous abortion, neonatal fatalities, lip and throat cancer, and other problems. An in the 1973 report, still another problem is highlighted—fetal and infant risks as consequences of smoking by pregnant women.[66]

- Some recent studies on smoke and other particulate inhalation show that environmental pollution may be a greater contributor to pulmonary disease and lung cancer than smoking. Although smoking is far from discounted as a factor, other things may be able to kill faster.[67]

- In the late 1800s, Pettenkofer linked health status with municipal water and sewage systems. Tuberculosis, cholera, and typhoid, among other diseases, were soon brought under control by simple sanitary expedients. In Munich, where Pettenkofer implemented his suggestions, the death rate from typhoid dropped from 150 deaths per year in 1871 to 14 in 1875.

- In 1962, Rachel Carson in *Silent Spring*[68] triggered widespread attention to the traces of organic pesticides now found in everyone alive on this planet. All of the potential disease implications are not yet known.

- Cholesterol levels in the human bloodstream derived from dietary habits have been linked with heart disease, although the exact relationship has not yet been explicated.[69]

- Studies of the impact of congestion on animals have been done and inferences drawn about both the physical and mental health of humans. Although little definitive knowledge has emerged, John Calhoun's investigations of rat behavior are disturbing. Under conditions of overcrowding, the rat colonies became, in his words, "behavioral sinks." Among the abnormalities Calhoun witnessed were bodily aggression; endocrinal disturbances, particularly affecting procreation; and cannibalism. One factor distinguishes Calhoun's research from other studies on congestion: in his experiments, the rats were given "space" in which to relieve the pressures of overcrowding, but they refused to disperse—their boundaries were psychological, not topographical.[70]

- The relationship between noise levels and health has been explored. Tentative results reveal that noise alters endocrinal, cardiovascular, and neurologic functions.[71] In one study, a higher rate of psychiatric admissions was associated with aircraft noise.[72] In his book *The Tyranny of Noise,* Robert Baron states:

> Noise, at even moderate levels, forces a systemic response from the total organism. It is not only the sense of hearing that is involved. What is also involved is what happens after the brain receives the sound signal. The brain places the body on a war footing. The repetition of these alerts is exhausting. It depletes energy levels in the volume of the blood circulation; it places a strain on the heart; it prevents restorative sleep and rest; it hinders

convalescence; it can be a form of torture. It can so weaken the body's defense mechanisms that diseases can more readily take hold. The organism does not adapt to noise; it becomes enured and pays a price. The price of this "adaptation" is in itself a hazard to health.[73]

Baron suggests that the frequency of sound waves is a possible explanation for much of the debilitation linked with noise. Certain sound-wave frequencies seem to be associated with illness in those exposed to the sound. As one example, Baron recounts Russian research that demonstrates irregularities in heart function in workers exposed to sound within the 85 and 120 decibel frequency.[74] Why else are signs posted outside hospitals instructing passersby to keep quiet?

- According to the U.S. Bureau of Community Environmental Management, 14,000 instances of rat bites were reported in 1970, together with 6000 cases of reported disease associated with rat infestation. And yet Congress refuses to implement effective rat control programs.

- Barry Commoner has estimated that radiation fallout has "probably caused about 5,000 defective births in the U.S. population and about 86,000 in the world population," up to 1963.[75] Other dangers associated with radiation include X-rays (how many children have been unnecessarily exposed to radiation in shoe stores through the use of portable X-ray machines?), thermal pollution from water used to cool nuclear reactors, and even airplanes.[76]

- A survey of vacationers at European beaches conducted by *Test-Achats,* a consumers' guide published in Europe, revealed that vacationers were twice as likely to contract a disease if they swam.[77] Many rivers in the United States, particularly the Ohio, the Potomac, and parts of the Missouri and Mississippi are equally dangerous. But natural waters are not the only problem. The water systems of Ames, Iowa; Evansville, Florida; Dade County, Florida; and Duluth, Minnesota have been found to contain dangerous chemical contaminants in amounts in excess of safe levels.[78]

- The effect of mercury ingestion on health has been relatively well established,[79] as has the impact of at least 4 of the 22 airborne metals that have been detected.[80]

- The findings of an 18-year study reflect a 32 percent increase in deaths from cancer among U.S. blacks, as opposed to an increase of only 3 percent for whites. Although the cause may be multifold, the report concludes that "greater exposure to environmental carcinogens must be suspected as the main cause for the faster increase of the black cancer mortality."[81]

- The greatest single predictor of longevity is not the fidelity of a patient to a physician, but job satisfaction. The amount of debilitation from job dissatisfaction is staggering.[82] This issue is taken up again later in this chapter.

- "Plumbism" is the catchy term used by physicians to refer to lead poisoning. This demonstrably preventable disease, contracted chiefly from exposure to lead-based paint on housing surfaces, affects from 10 to 25 percent of children who live in urban slums. Of these, 2 to 5 percent have the signs of poisoning, which leads to permanent brain damage.[83]

- The consumption of a large amount of coffee may be linked with heart disease.[84]

- Finally, in a comprehensive review of the literature on the relationship between air pollution and human health, Lave and Seskin state:

The studies show a close association between air pollution and ill health. The evidence is extremely good for some diseases (such as bronchitis and lung cancer) and only suggestive for others (such as cardiovascular disease and nonrespiratory-tract cancers). . .

Lave and Seskin go on to draw some specific implications for health. They conclude that mortality from bronchitis would be lowered by roughly 50 percent if air pollution were lowered to levels currently prevailing in urban areas with relatively clean air. As to lung cancer, approximately 25 percent of the mortality could be avoided by a 50 percent reduction in air pollution. The price we pay in poor health is about $33 million per year.

According to Lave and Seskin, the studies also show relationships between all respiratory diseases and air pollution. About 25 percent of all morbidity and mortality due to respiratory disease could be eliminated by a 50 percent abatement in air pollution. Since the annual cost of respiratory disease is $4887 million, the amount saved by a 50 percent reduction in air pollution in major urban areas would be $1222 million. Of course, estimates of savings can be misleading. It is true that resources might be saved if the programs suggested by Lave and Seskin were implemented. But to estimate the actual savings, the additional costs of establishing the programs must be added to the calculation.

There is also evidence that over 20 percent of the deaths due to cardiovascular disorders could be avoided if air pollution were reduced by 50 percent. The savings might be $468 million per year. Finally, Lave and Seskin point to evidence connecting all mortality from cancer with air pollution; they then estimate that 15 percent of the costs of cancer could be saved by a 50 percent reduction in air pollution—or a total of $390 million per year.[85]

Lave and Seskin's work is corroborated by research done by Ronald Ridken. Ridken estimates, very conservatively, that 18 to 20 percent of the roughly $2 billion spent on treatment of respiratory diseases could be "saved" if the quality of air was improved.[86]

On top of these dangers, there will be deferred effects. To quote Dubos again:

It is probable that continued exposure to low levels of toxic agents will eventually result in a great variety of delayed pathological manifestations, creating more physiological misery and increasing the medical load. The point of importance here is that the worst pathological effects of environmental pollutants will *not* be detected at the time of exposure; indeed they may not become evident *until several decades later.* In other words, society will become adjusted to levels of pollution sufficiently low not to have an immediate nuisance value, but this apparent adaptation will eventually cause much pathological damage in the adult population and create large medical and social burdens.[87]

MENTAL AND EMOTIONAL DISORDER

In 1962, the results of the Midtown Manhattan study were announced.[88] Among the findings was that the degree of psychiatric disorder in the institutionalized population, that is, those under treatment, was matched in the general population.

The Midtown study is one of many studies seeking to peg the degree of mental illness in the population, as distinguished from examination of institutionalized populations.[89] These studies, which are generally referred to as psychiatric epidemiology research, ostensibly establish a baseline from which relative levels of mental and emotional disorder can be determined. However, there are two severe limitations. The first is, assuming that a baseline can be fixed, in the words of three investigators, Cooper, Fry, and Kalton, that "there has been a dearth of longitudinal studies of psychiatric illness in the community."[90] This lack, of course, makes it difficult to measure levels of mental illness over time. A study undertaken by Cooper et al. attempted a remedy— 4000 patients were followed for seven years. Seven years is probably not sufficient to permit inferences about long-term trends, but the study revealed that mean prevalence rates of psychiatric disorder over the seven-year period were consistently higher than at the beginning of the project.

The second limitation arises from problems with definition and classification. The classic studies—the Midtown work, the study of New Haven by Hollingshead and Redlich, the Lemkau et al. work in Baltimore, and Alexander Leighton's research in Nova Scotia—conflict. Their findings show a disparity of 8 per 1000 to 815 per 1000 cases of "mental illness."[91] Much of this variation is undoubtedly due to varying definitions of "mental illness." Unfortunately, psychometric testing, which could generate harder numbers, is apparently too embryonic. Reliance on institutional census data is also misplaced. In Minnesota, for example, the census in state hospitals has fallen from a peak of 11,800 persons to 2400 in 1972. This neither means the Minnesotans are more healthy, nor that the incidence of mental illness generally is decreasing. Rather, the figures can be explained as the result of the initiation of community-based treatment programs and the shift of many aged persons to long-term care facilities.

The theory is conflicting as well. Harvey Wheeler, a Senior Fellow at the Center for the Study of Democratic Institutions, in an unpublished paper, "The Morbid Society," offers an argument that mental illness is increasing. His argument rests on some untested premises: that modern society preserves its defectives; that the nuclear (or "molecular," to use his term) family breeds mental illness in a kind of cybernetic way through mutual adaptations to pathology in one member; and, finally, that the idleness of the young through deferred "rites of passage" induces neurosis. He concludes that "contemporary America may be the first society in history to be composed almost entirely of emotionally disturbed persons." If Wheeler is right, things will not get any better by the year 2000.

Some of the other arguments supporting the proposition that mental illness is increasing are analogous to those marshalled to demonstrate increases in cardiovascular disease: more stress, more congestion, more domestic strife, more and faster change, and so on. And there are some data relating these conditions and morbidity. Some studies, referred to earlier, have established linkages between critical life events, such as marriage, divorce, loss of job, and so on, and the onset of illness.[92]

A final line of argument is offered principally by ethnologists and anthropologists, including Lionel Tiger, Desmond Morris, Robert Ardrey, and Konrad Lorenz.[93] A common feature of their thinking is that inherent defects exist in our genetic machinery which lead to aberrant and possibly destructive behavior. Lorenz amplifies his thinking in his latest book, *Civilized Man's Eight Deadly Sins.*[94] Arthur Koestler stakes out some of the same ground in *The Ghost in the Machine.*[95] In Koestler's view, an inherent defect, the ghost in the machine, may cause man to destroy himself. None of these theories attempts to peg specific levels of mental illness. Rather, in all cases the forecast is that the deficiencies coded into the human species will play themselves out in ensuing years.

Srole is more optimistic in his analysis of the Midtown findings:

> If we were required to venture a probability estimate of the mental health consequences (of our examination in "Midtown"), we would offer this as our most general extrapolation: weighing the primary gains and secondary effects . . . suggests a likely net effect of large-scale *improvement* in the overall mental health composition of the American population.[96]

In part, Srole premises the extrapolation on the easing of conditions which presumably contribute to high levels of mental illness. He states:

> With these massive humane gains have come a number of secondary side effects, including psychological strains inherent

in adapting to rapid change, tensions generated by the heightened insecurity and competitiveness of a more fluid status
system, erosions in the doctrinal and moral areas of the religious sphere, and loosening in the cathected qualities and sup-
portiveness of interpersonal relations. To this incomplete list
might be added extension of the concept of machine and
product obsolescence toward economic and social devaluation
of the aged.[97]

It is doubtful, however, that the conditions he recites
either have abated or will abate. But there are other arguments. Goldhammer and Marshall, in *Psychosis and Civilization*,[98] after tracing mental hospital admission rates in
Massachusetts in the nineteenth century, and controlling for
classes of patients and conditions affecting hospitalization of
the mentally ill, found that "admissions rates for ages under
80 [were] just as high . . . as they are today."[99] The study was
limited to admission rates, and given the flexibility of admission policies the study does not refute the argument that
modern man suffers more mental derangement. Many factors govern hospitalization. Moreover, institutionalization is
not synonymous with mental illness.

Other research suggests that some mental illness is a function of social and economic status. Recent work by Dohrenwend and Dohrenwend, reported in *Social Status and
Psychological Disorder*,[100] offers this argument. In combination with Goldhammer and Marshall's work, their report
casts further doubt on the proposition that mental illness is
increasing.

Analysis of this subject butts up against three constraints.
The first is the lack of a paradigm in psychology. Until a
cohesive theory of human behavior emerges, if ever, all
investigation will be complicated by definitional warfare. Of
course, some theories have been offered as paradigms; the
hotly and widely disputed B. F. Skinner has offered a
hypothesis, for example.[101] In oversimplified terms, Skinner
argues that behavior conforms to and can be explained by
the effects of positive and aversive reinforcement in a system

of constant and mutual feedback between the individual and the environment. Skinner, so far as I know, has not directly addressed the degree of pathology in the population, but his work is consistent with the view that mental illness will increase. If the culture we create sets the parameters for conditioning, and if culture is increasingly being created by persons who are mentally ill, it follows that a disordered environment will foster mental and emotional disorder to the same or even greater degree.

The second constraint relates to efficacy. Mental health is a swamp of uncertain dimensions. Some therapeutic regimes work for some patients, but it is hard to isolate any constants. Some operant conditioning techniques applied in limited and controlled settings such as school classrooms and some mental health institutions have been successfully demonstrated. Success is also reported by some psychoanalysts. Finally, psychoactive drugs, while controversial, apparently work in some settings.[102] But there is little hard research, despite voluminous evidence. Robert Coles, a Harvard psychoanalyst, states the difficulty nicely: "We are in a world of feeling, the doctor's as much as the patient's, so no amount of training or credentials or reputation can remove the hazards of such a world."[103] Eli Ginzberg, an observer of health affairs, builds on Coles's assertion:

Many articulate psychiatrists have reportedly testified before Congress about significant therapeutic advances. But we must question whether there is solid evidence, reinforced by follow-up to support such claims. Admittedly, state hospital census figures are down, not up; yet there has been an upward drift in patient admissions figures. But the total system has been changing and we now treat many patients in new kinds of settings. Are they included in the totals? Another reason for caution is the readmissions rate. Still another is what happens to the patient who is discharged. Is his recovery maintained? Not much is known. To release a patient from the hospital is easier than to absorb him at home. And without adequate follow-up data, we remain in the dark.[104]

A third constraint is that definitions of deviance are relative; they change over time. Kai Erikson in *Wayward Pilgrims*[105] traced the shifts in definitions of deviance underlying attitudes and values toward it in Puritan Massachusetts. From roughly 1650 to 1655, the citizens of Salem were sufficiently exercised to label fornication, drunkenness, and vagrancy as deviant acts. Then for about 15 years, from 1655 to 1670, they shifted to punishing "witches." When all of the witches had either been destroyed or converted, from roughly 1670 to 1680, the Salem citizenry once again became bothered by fornication, drunkenness, and vagrancy. But despite radical changes in the definitions of deviance, the supply of deviants remained roughly constant.

Some of this same slippage in definitions can be observed today. In recent decades, the definitions of certain behaviors have blurred—abortion and drug use to name but two. These activities, long considered as crimes, are being reevaluated. The result may be decriminalization. As long as deviance is a relative quality, it is difficult to conceive of the mental health system as anything other than society's choice of mechanisms to police behavior that is considered offensive. This conclusion is not unique. Thomas Szasz and R. D. Laing, both therapists, have argued along these lines.[106]

Three recent studies sum up my points. In the first, a group of eight college students and teachers postured as deranged persons in search of asylum. Each was readily admitted to an institution. After resuming "normal" behavior, they were nevertheless undetected by the staffs. The only people who caught on were the other patients. In each case, the researchers recorded their experiences. At discharge, which averaged 19 days from admission, each was diagnosed as a schizophrenic in remission.[107] (As an intriguing sidelight, 2100 pills were administered to them during their captivity.)

The second example, a cross-cultural study, reflects the universality of therapy.[108] The common therapies utilized by therapists include drug therapy, shock therapy, dream analysis, and conditioning techniques. (One measure employed in Nigeria, which must be categorized as aversive operant conditioning, is too good to pass up. Bedwetters in Nigeria, it seems, are treated by tying a toad to the male child's penis. When the child wets, the toad croaks and the child wakes up. There are two difficulties with the method: first, it fails to solve the problem of female bedwetting. Second, it asks a lot of the toads.)

In most major cities, the "high-rise" building is the collective badge of distinction. At the same time, the high-rise may be socially disintegrative. Oscar Newman, an architect at New York University, found that the crime rate increased almost proportionately with building height in low-income housing projects.[109] These conclusions are buttressed by Greek architect and city planner, Constantine Doxiadis, who acknowledges in an article, "Confessions of a Criminal," that his most heinous "crime" was to have advocated high-rise buildings. He explains:

> Such buildings work against nature by spoiling the scale of the landscape. The most successful cities of the past have been the ones where man and his buildings were in a certain balance with nature, such as Athens or Florence. [High-rise] buildings work against man himself, especially against children who lose their direct contacts with nature. Even where the contact is maintained, it is subject to parental control. As a result, the children suffer and so do the parents. Furthermore, these buildings work against society because they do not help the units of social importance—the family and the extended family, the neighborhood—to function as naturally and as normally as before.[110]

What does this research combine to say? The lesson of the first is that labeling, while relative and often grossly inaccurate, can be viciously destructive as well. It is difficult, given the current state of the art, to determine who needs treatment and who does not; many of those under treatment may simply be there fortuitously. Yet treatment is dished out every day under the banner of science.

If the first study demonstrates relativity, the second demonstrates universality. Certain therapeutic techniques are common to many cultures. They are rooted in the history of the species and manifest themselves in many different ways in widely differing cultures. We cannot assume that treatment in contemporary Western civilization is more efficacious simply because it appears to be more sophisticated.

Third and finally, mental health services emphasize cures, not causes. Why is it that architects are writing about high-rise buildings? A better example is the relationship between poverty and mental health. Matthew Dumont asserts in *The Absurd Healer*,[111] an examination of community mental health, that "study after study has demonstrated the relationship between poverty and mental illness."[112] If this is so, more mental health professionals should get into the trenches and try to find out what causes mental illness, and when they find out, as in the case of poverty, face the dilemma of dealing with causes or massaging symptoms. Until more do so, mental health treatment may not go much further than tying toads to penises.

BREAKTHROUGHS IN BIOMEDICAL TECHNOLOGY

Both futurologists and biomedical researchers have made predictions about potential technological breakthroughs. The futurologists Kahn and Weiner include among their list of "one hundred technical innovations likely in the next thirty-three years" the following biomedical speculations:[113]

- major reduction in hereditary and congenital defects;
- extensive use of cyborg techniques;
- controlled, supereffective relaxation and sleep therapies;

- new, more varied, and more reliable drugs for control of fatigue, relaxation, alertness, mood, personality, perceptions, and fantasies;
- general and substantial increase in life expectancy, postponement of aging, and limited rejuvenation;
- high quality medical care for underdeveloped areas;
- more extensive use of transplantation of human organs;
- widespread use of cryogenics or freezing techniques;
- improved chemical control of some mental illness and some aspects of senility; and
- extensive genetic control for plants and animals.

In *The Biological Time Bomb,* Gordon Rattray Taylor formulated a "Table of Developments":

Phase One: by 1975
Extensive transplantation of limbs and organs
Test-tube fertilization of human eggs
Implantation of fertilized eggs in womb
Indefinite storage of eggs and spermatozoa
Choice of sex of offspring
Extensive power to postpone clinical death
Mind-modifying drugs: regulation of desire
Memory erasure
Imperfect artificial placenta
Artificial viruses

Phase Two: by 2000
Extensive mind modification and personality reconstruction
Enhancement of intelligence in men and animals
Memory injection and memory editing
Perfected artificial placenta and true baby factory
Life-copying—reconstructed organisms
Hibernation and prolonged coma
Prolongation of youthful vigor
First cloned animals
Synthesis of unicellular organisms
Organ regeneration
Man-animal chimeras

Phase Three: after 2000

Control of aging: extension of life span
Synthesis of complex living organisms
Disembodied brains
Brain-computer links
Gene insertion and deletion
Cloned people
Brain-brain links
Man-machine chimeras
Indefinite postponement of death[114]

Helmer and de Brigard included the following list in their work, "Some Potential Societal Developments, 1970–2000":[115]

    a. The development of non-narcotic personality drugs;
    b. Mass administered contraceptives;
    c. The ability to choose the sex of offspring;
    d. General immunization agents;
    e. Intelligence drugs; and
    f. Some degree of control over hereditary defects.

Whether all of this will occur is problematic. However, given the level of research and development expenditures in the biomedical field, some breakthroughs will undoubtedly be made. Federal support increased from $50 million in 1940 to $1.2 billion in 1965, and has continued to grow, although it was blunted by the Nixon Administration. Nonetheless, 1972 budgetary allocations for the National Institute of Health and the National Institute of Mental Health were $1,143,202 and $144,668,000 respectively.[116] And those figures do not include sums allocated to the "crusade against cancer," which were expected to reach $1 billion a year by 1975.

Attitudes toward biomedical research may, however, affect the amount of resources available. There is increasing skepticism about the capacity of science and technology to make life better. If doubts continue, biomedical technology may be among the first areas to suffer. An undercurrent of skepticism about research on the functioning of the human animal, particularly human genetic constitution and reproductive capacities, has always existed. Reports about "test-tube babies" exercise more people than reports about "The Green Revolution." Nevertheless, many of the breakthroughs forecast for the human species focus on reproduction and the genetic structure. On the other hand, skepticism about science is mostly directed at the hard physical sciences. Pollution triggers much of it—the technology derived from advances in the physical sciences can be traced as the cause of environmental degradation. Biomedical advances (except for the noxious practices of chemical and biological warfare), seem, by contrast, to offer more varied and rich life experiences.

If attitudes toward science and technology do not dramatically harden, and if funding for biomedical research does not dry up, society is clearly on the threshold of major breakthroughs that create the potential for development of a far more sophisticated medical care system. This may bring mixed results. But in any event, what kind of breakthroughs can be expected?[117]

Thirty years ago, biology was a relatively simple science that focused on the reproductive capacities of fruit flies and the behavior of molds. The nature of the genes was a mystery, the structure of DNA unimagined, the functions of RNA unknown. The means of protein synthesis were not understood and the replication of viruses was an enigma. Powerful drugs like streptomycine, chlorpromazine, and the use of DDT and LSD lay in the future. Even the hardware was crude. Isotopes were rare and costly, centrifuges and oscilloscopes were clumsy, and the electron microscope was restricted in its application, as were the phase microscope, the transistor, the computer, the laser, and holography. Invention and implementation of this technology over the last 30 years has enriched the biological knowledge available to medicine.

Based on what has been done and work in progress, what are the areas of biological science that hold promise?

MOLECULAR THERAPY. At present, chemical intervention into biological systems relies upon the introduction of small molecules like penicillin and cortisone. Within the next 30 years, large and complex molecular proteins, nuclear acids, and even viruses may be developed. And knowledge of cellular biology should advance sufficiently to permit use of such molecules in therapy.

IMMUNE REJECTION. The development of refined therapies depends on the means to harness and control immune rejection. Our understanding of immune rejection has rapidly advanced but is not yet complete. However, advances within a decade may establish a tolerance for specific therapies. Present methods deal with rejection by virtually destroying the entire immune system. Once immune tolerance is achieved, molecular agents might be designed to interfere with viral assembly and replication. The result might be increasing control of viral diseases, including the so-called "slow viruses," which are suspected by some as the cause of many debilitative and degenerative conditions.

TRANSPLANTS. Tolerance by the human organism will also enhance surgical transplantation. Transplantation of organs such as the kidneys, the heart, the liver, and the lungs is now feasible, although results are mixed. But widespread use of transplants is limited by the intractability of immune rejection. Dr. Robert Sinsheimer of the California Institute of Technology believes that a solution to the rejection problem might make treatment possible for the approximately 20,000 to 30,000 heart transplant candidates per year, and for another 7500 kidney transplants. This is a vivid example of medicine for the few—even if they number in the thousands.[118]

Transplantation in the future may also include xenography, that is, the transplantation of primate or cattle organs into human beings. The use of xenografts may be necessary because of an insufficient number of human donors.

Acceleration of transplant techniques could also occur if artificial organs are developed over the next 30 years. Questions about the relative merits of artificial versus natural organs cannot be answered at this time. But the development and implementation of artificial organs seems possible within the next 30 years.

PROSTHETIC DEVICES. A marked advance in the quality and sophistication of prosthesis is expected. New technology will even aid those with impaired vision.

GENETIC AND POPULATION PROBLEMS. Some of the most difficult value questions arise in this area. Even though childbirth rates are declining in advanced countries, population pressures continue in the world. Even the United States will experience an absolute increase in population. A difficult issue arises when techniques are developed that enhance the likelihood of the survival of persons who would otherwise succumb to hereditary and genetic defects. In some cases, when genetic controls are available, attitides toward their use may result in their suppression. For example, amniocentisis for the detection of genetic defects in the uterus is possible and effective. But controversy swirls around its use.[119] Other breakthroughs expected include further development of sperm banks and the development of cloning tissue banks. Moreover, *in vitro* human fertilization followed by implantation in a natural or foster mother will likely become feasible within 30 years.[120]

DRUGS AND THE MIND. Advances in neurobiology and psychopharmacology will lead to the discovery of new and powerful mind-altering drugs. Some of the drugs will make it possible to enhance memory and even to improve intelligence. Related technologies such as implantation of electrodes to stimulate centers in the brain or relieve hormonal or epileptic conditions are also feasible.

SOPHISTICATED TECHNOLOGY AND SYSTEMS ANALYSIS. Development of the means of intervention in the biological system, when combined with the techniques of systems analysis, may accelerate the use of highly sophisticated methods for treatment of diseases which resist any single therapy. Thus, for example, a combination of chemotherapy and radiation therapy might have far-reaching effects in the treatment of a cancer when the use of only one of the therapies hits a brick wall. Systems analysis facilitates the coordinated use of more than one therapy at a time. Among other things this should lead to better therapies to treat hormonal problems and cardiovascular diseases. Ultimately, even the aging process may be attacked through a combination of therapies, leavened by systems analysis.

Medicine has been able to build upon sturdy biomedical foundations in the last few decades. And more biomedical breakthroughs are expected. Many can and will be implemented in medical care. But biomedical innovation is not necessarily an unmitigated good—there is another perspective.

The overall physician to population ratio for the United States is approximately 1:670. The prevailing physician-patient ratio for kidney dialysis is 1:2; for coronary care units it is roughly 1:10. Both therapies are recent biomedical engineering breakthroughs. In some underserved parts of the country, the physician-patient ratio is as high as 1:10,000 persons. Kidney dialysis and coronary care units (CCU's), while costly and complicated, do save lives. But estimates for the cost of kidney dialysis alone are pegged at $1 billion per year within 10 years; roughly $135 million was spent in

1972.[121] These treatments for heart and kidney disease are two instances where the impact of medical practice is demonstrable. What about the CCU, then?

In 1969, the Commission on Professional and Hospital Activities compared the effectiveness of sample hospitals with and without coronary care units. The study revealed that 25.7 percent of the 54,506 myocardial infarction patients admitted to all the participating hospitals died, but only 20.7 percent of patients treated in CCU's died, contrasted with 27.7 percent of patients who did not receive CCU treatment. In this study, then, 2700 more persons might have survived if CCU treatment had been used in all cases.[122] There is contrary evidence. A British study referred to earlier revealed no significant differences in either morbidity or mortality in patients treated at home or in the hospital. But let us assume that CCU's save lives.[123]

The cost of installation and maintenance of a CCU in an existing hospital is about $30,000 per bed per year. The number of patients who can be treated in one CCU in one year (assuming 80 percent occupancy) is about 45. Using the Commission figures, .05 patients in one year might be saved in the average CCU bed at the cost of $30,000. And if each of the 7000 hospitals in the United States had 10 CCU beds, 35,000 patients might be saved annually at a cost of about $2.5 billion, or about $70,000 per patient saved. This illustrates the astronomical costs of care even when the system works. As Anne Somers has said, "The more advanced and the more effective the technology, the greater the overall costs of care."[124] But the CCU illustration suggests two other propositions. The first is the interest of the system in the sophisticated, however effective. Many of today's physicians seem to be frustrated engineers. The style of medical practice ineluctably follows the development of new technology.

Second, it illuminates some of the trade offs in medicine that are rarely considered. The cost-effectiveness ratio (with effectiveness expressed only as lives saved) of CCU's (assuming the rough accuracy of the figures above) is about one life for $70,000. This is about the salary of two physicians delivering care to an area without medical care resources. Further, based on some recent cost-benefit research recited in an article[125] by Robert Grosse, the expenditure of only $2200 would prevent one death from cervical cancer. More strikingly, maternal and child health programs—examples of effective prevention programs—for an expenditure of $10 million would have the benefits depicted in Figure 12.

If CCU's were discontinued and the savings plowed into these programs, 250 maternal and child health programs could be established.

Yet another example is emergency health. Dr. Robert Huntley, then head of the Health Service Division of Emergency Health Services, argued that "we can save lives with adequately equipped ambulances and properly trained personnel. It may be 50,000, or 75,000, but a figure of 60,000 is in the right ball park."[126] The costs of emergency care are paltry in comparison; .002 of the national medical care budget is allocated to emergency care, lack of which kills more persons in this country under age 37 than *any* other cause.[127]

Kidney dialysis poses the same issues. According to recent cost estimates, 5000 dialysis patients, the projected number of users by 1985, will *each* consume $200,000 per year, for a total of $1 billion per year.[128] If we took the same amount of money—the savings from not deploying dialysis units—and placed it into, for example, pollution control, or programs of mass transit, or any number of other programs which remove or abate conditions that cause ill health, the overall impact on health, while difficult to calculate, might be substantially greater.

Calculations of reductions in mortality and morbidity resulting from preventive programs are necessarily crude, and also encumbered with value judgments. But one thing is clear—we are utilizing CCU's and kidney dialysis units for

FIGURE 12 YEARLY EFFECTS PER $10,000,000 EXPENDED IN HEALTH-DEPRESSED AREAS

	Comprehensive Programs		Case Finding of Treatment 0, 1, 3, 5, 7, 9 Years of Age
	To Age 18	To Age 5	
Maternal deaths prevented	1.6	3	
Premature births prevented	100–250	200–485	
Infant deaths prevented	40–60	85–120	
Mental retardation prevented	5–7	7–14	
Handicaps prevented or corrected by age 18:			
Vision problems: All	350	195	3470
Amblyopia	60	119	1140
Hearing loss: All	90	70	7290
Binaural	6	5	60
Other physical handicap	200	63	1470

Source. Robert Grosse, "Cost Benefit Analysis of Health Service," *The Annals of the American Academy of Political and Social Science*, **399** (January 1972), 98.

patients who can afford them, or who are eligible for public
support, but we are not providing care to underserved areas,
and we are not attacking the causes of sickness. The point is
not that CCU's and kidney dialysis do not save lives, but
rather that the decision to save lives of those patients who
suffer myocardial infarction or renal failure is made by a
system that has not or will not consider other ways to save
other lives and possibly more lives at less cost.

By the year 2000, if biomedical breakthroughs comparable
to kidney dialysis and the CCU are made, medical care costs
will rise even more rapidly, roughly commensurate with the
costs of the new technology. Medical practice will become
even more highly specialized. And finally, if a treatment
orientation continues to dominate medicine, the opportunity
to subject the trade offs between various alternative medical
care expenditures to public debate will be no greater than it
is now. Preventive programs will continue to be starved.

THE CRISIS IN SERVICE INSTITUTIONS[129]

Today manufactured goods account for little more than 25
percent of the gross national product. Shortly, perhaps
within a quarter of a century, this proportion will decline to
less than 10 percent. The remainder of the GNP will be
accounted for by services, which include everything from
practicing law to running TWA to serving fast foods. But
the major expansion is expected in "well-being" services
—medical care, education, and welfare and social services.
In other words, material commodities will be overrun by
well-being commodities; our pursuit of well-being may dis-
place our acquisition of material goods. If this occurs, welfare, education, and medical care may take on the characteristics of capital items. Society must then face questions
about well-being that were faced in the past about material
commodities.

In the past, a key question was how to guarantee all citizens at least subsistence. The question in the future will increasingly become how to guarantee the rights of all citizens to well-being. This analysis is consistent with Abraham Maslow's theory of "basic needs."[130] To Maslow, there is a "hierarchy" of needs which man, and derivatively his culture and polity, must pursue. The first and most basic is physiological; next come safety needs; third, belongingness and love; and finally, self-actualization. The latter concept corresponds with the idea of well-being.

In terms of politics, government, having addressed itself (without necessarily succeeding) to the physiological and safety needs, will turn to ensuring opportunities for self-actualization. In part, human services spring from this idea. Day-care and child-care programs are often based on the self-actualization needs of mothers. Most contemporary welfare reform proposals at least implicitly owe some allegiance to this idea.

The by-product of governmental response to self-actualization needs is the growth of service bureaucracies. If well-being is a scarce commodity, which is a plausible assumption, it is a new kind of scarcity. In the past, many commodities were scarce. Society sought to alleviate scarcity by correcting inequities in income distribution and by attacking the industrial monopolists' control of the market. However, well-being can only be scarce when its delivery is constrained by bureaucracies and by providers. This will lead to consideration of a problem realized in the collectivist democracies many years ago. Monopolization of authority by bureaucrats led to the creation of an official elite, which in turn discriminated against those less entrenched in the bureaucracy or those outside. The same kind of rigidities and discriminations might appear in the United States as it changes from an industrial to a service economy. If so, change from a subsistence to a well-being society will be accompanied by a struggle against different injustices. The phenomenon is already perceivable. Service sectors often pursue internal objectives in derogation of the public interest. The slow strangulation of New York City by those in control of vital services—fire, police, sanitation—is a good example.

And if all of this is so, a series of severe social, political, and organizational problems may erupt. Well-being services are produced by the great provider institutions: law, medicine, government, and so on. However, all these systems are in severe disarray and under strong pressure to change. At the very time we are moving from a manufacturing to a service economy, the major service systems are in a state of crisis analogous to that suffered by manufacturing industries in the 1920s and 1930s. A remedy for the crisis in medical services is being sought through federal financing—a national health insurance plan. The assumption is that governmental absorption of the costs of care will redress access and distributional inequities. If a national health insurance plan is enacted, some of the inequities may be curbed or modulated. But the price will be high. The underlying premise of medical care financing reform is that medicine produces enough health to justify the enormous expenditure. This is not the case, but there are other dangers as well.

A larger governmental role, particularly through financing, will strengthen and intensify professionalism in medicine, not weaken it as many providers have argued. The reason is simple. A national health insurance plan will specify that only professional services can be bought. Consumers with cash can buy virtually any service from any person or agency willing to sell it, subject only to the loose strictures of state licensing and certification laws. But with federal assumption of the costs of care, the care that can be bought will inevitably be the care that is already provided. This might not be an unhappy result if professionalization in medicine were an unvarnished good. But the goals of professionals are rarely the same as the goals of those whom they serve.

Professionalized service bureaucracies—health, education, police, fire, transport, and so forth—are not as responsive as most of us think they should be. As services become professionalized, as most have, the service bureaucracy becomes less sensitive to social needs and more impervious to social controls. Few have questioned the need for each judge to have a private bathroom in chambers, nor the physician's "right" to work when and how he or she wishes. More will question the sanitary workers when they allow garbage to pile up on the streets. The more the public becomes subservient to the professional, and the less the consumer gets for more money, the more will the public's sense of helplessness grow.

As government assumes the responsibility for the financing of medical care, it will necessarily install a large bureaucracy to police the flow of public funds into private hands. Concomitantly, it will expand its regulatory apparatus to scrutinize the quality of the product it is buying, the means by which it is provided, and the distribution of the resources it is creating. If these bureaucracies behave as other service bureaucracies have—and there is no reason to assume otherwise—they will impede rather than facilitate the flow of benefits from providers to consumers. But paradoxically, they will also seek to preserve the flow of benefits from providers to consumers. Jobs will depend on the maintenance of the service system as it is. The entrenchment of a bureaucracy that feeds off a service by serving as an intermediary between provider and consumer will then frustrate if not prevent change in the service system of the future.

But there is even a greater danger. As the government assumes larger obligations for services and as the economy gradually shifts to a service economy, bureaucracies will swell in power as well as size. In the past, a key problem has been the rapacity of the private sector which controlled the resources necessary for a decent life. But in the future, control over the flow of resources will rest more with bureaucracies and bureaucrats. Evidence is available that medical care has less impact on health than a variety of other factors. The growth and strength of service bureaucracies will frustrate attempts to reallocate resources—to shift resources from services to other programs with a potentially greater impact on health.

THE COMPUTER REVOLUTION: THE HIGH TECHNOLOGY OF THE FUTURE

The computer revolution will continue in the next 30 years. Today's computers are already deployed in medical care; scores of software salesmen visit doctors' offices and hospital corridors. The computer, one example of high medical technology, can improve medical care, but there are hazards as well.

DECISION-MAKING. Decisions regarding the kind and the amount of medical care are made by the physician, but also to an increasing extent by government. The consumer has the least say in these decisions. Currently, federal and state governments together purchase about 40 percent of the medical care provided in this country.[131] The computer, however, might make the democratic process more participatory. Referenda could be held through the use of computer-assisted polling procedures. This could result in an enlarged role for consumers of medical care. However, it is equally possible that the computer will facilitate despotic manipulation of consumers; it could dramatically lessen consumers' opportunities to affect decisions about health care services. Consumers know even less about computers than they know about medical care.

There is one promising development. The computer might make possible instantaneous interaction between patient and provider without the necessity of an office or hospital visit. For example, a person experiencing certain symptoms may be able to take advantage of a computer link with a physician's office. A computer could be utilized for interrogation of the patient and instantaneous coding of the patient responses. This is an example of how medical care might be made more accessible to the consumer.

THE INCREASING SOPHISTICATION OF CARE. Medical care has steadily become more sophisticated. Greater use of the computer in the provision of care will accelerate this trend. The use of the computer in triage—situations in which decisions must be made as to who will receive life-saving medical care—has occurred. In a hospital in Salt Lake City, Utah, that is almost entirely computerized, use of the computer system presumably makes a physician's diagnosis more accurate. Reliance on the computer will undoubtedly increase markedly in the next 20 to 30 years.

Another product of further development of computer technology is the patient computer console. Patients could be provided with home consoles that would be programmed with information relating to their own condition and past treatment, and perhaps linked with the physician's computer system. Through use of the console, patients would be able to retrieve information relating to their conditions almost instantaneously. The potential for self-care is obvious. Since they pose an obvious threat to professional prerogatives, providers will probably resist the use of home consoles.

One potentially adverse consequence of increased use of the computer in medical care derives from the fact that computers cost money. Widespread deployment of computers will drive up the costs of care and foster further specialization. The recent history of medical care reflects the unabating sophistication of medical care technology and the rapid specialization of practitioners. As more sophisticated technology is implemented, substantial numbers of citizens will be deprived of care which only the rich will be able to afford. The alternative is the subsidy of costly procedures under a national health insurance program. But limits on the public purse will soon be reached, and a private market for the most costly procedures will undoubtedly develop.

IMPACT ON THE PHYSICIAN. One of the dualities in medicine referred to in Chapter 3 is the schism between the anthropologic and technical approaches to care. If future use of the computer is dictated by the proponents of technical care, an even greater erosion in the anthropologic approach can be expected. The computer is a machine. When intelligently used by the physician and the patient, the computer might lead to more accuracy in both diagnosis and treatment. The question, however, is what the cost of this accuracy may be. Further deemphasis in the human or anthropologic approach may have unforeseen costs that far outweigh the benefits of the use of the computer. The prognosis for the anthropologic model of medical care is not good. The computer, as one of the most powerful and alluring tools for technicians, will contribute to its demise.

IMPACT ON THE PATIENT. The alienation of individuals when grappling with large and complex organizations is conveyed in an extensive literature. The scale and complexity of the medical care system have important implications for health. There is no definitive evidence correlating health with the scale of the treatment system, but the scale of the delivery system is growing, irrespective of the means taken to finance care, or the nature of structural reforms within the system. Increasing sophistication of the medical hardware and superspecialization by practitioners has led to larger units for the delivery of care. How else can comprehensive care be provided? But impersonality is a concomitant of increased size. Since the computer increases the potential for control of larger and more complex operations and feeds the specialization craze, more extensive use of the computer will facilitate the evolution of larger and more complex units for care.

Increases in the size of institutions further attenuates the patient's responsibility for health. Historically, with the rise of the professions of health, the individual has been relieved of responsibility for health. The advent of larger systems of care will force already dependent patients to relate to bricks, mortar, and bureaucrats. In the past their dependence was at least upon flesh and blood. Something in the relationship between patient and physician may be essential to the patient's well-being.

WORK

In 1972, the Department of Health, Education and Welfare issued a report entitled *Work in America*.[132] Unlike most government reports, its language was blunt: workers in the United States dislike what they do, in some cases intensely. In addition to apathy, there has also been an increase in work-related injuries, in sabotage, and in defects in workmanship.[133] The Bureau of Labor Statistics reports an increase in the number of disabling work-related injuries from 11.8 per million employees in 1961 to 15.2 in 1970.[134] There are also hosts of occupational diseases. Among these are black-lung disease, silicosis, and asbestos and lead poisoning.[135]

Then there is stress. Some features of stress and its relationship to health are related to work habits and practices. The stress associated with the role of the upper middle class businessman and professional has received attention, perhaps more than the data merit. There is no doubt that the competitiveness and drive that characterize the ambitious businessman and professional drain resources otherwise put to health. Moreover, the social and ethical concomitants of success —dinner and cocktail parties, and long, liquid lunches, undoubtedly contribute to the deterioration of health among those who have chosen, or who are compulsively driven, to become leaders in commerce and business.

But the health problems of those who cannot afford long lunch hours and cocktail parties are often overlooked, and may be more severe. From 1947 to 1962, man-hour productivity in nonfarm, unskilled labor increased 60 percent; in agriculture the increase was 242 percent. But the work week was not shortened. Given the added hours of commuting to the job, for many the actual work week has increased. This results in what one investigator has referred to as "work-stress syndrome":

> A work-stress syndrome may be postulated which is applicable to a wide variety of current American occupations—manufacturing operatives, clerical workers, technicians and others. This syndrome includes large-muscle immobilization, severe, protracted, time-sensory-motion discipline, high noise and vibration levels, and intense illumination. It is often aggravated by anxiety: random dangers and needs for immediate response associated with traffic hazards in commuting; underlying anxieties associated with the obsolescence of the worker's skills and need for constant retraining.[136]

All this can lead to poor health. Whether conditions will worsen over the next few decades is problematic. There is a strong argument that stress related to employment will increase. But at the same time, a shift to a service economy and proposed reduction in the work week might offset some of the stress. In any event, it is doubtful that the "work-stress syndrome" will disappear.

POVERTY AND HEALTH

The subject of poverty and health deserves a treatise; I can give it only a moment of reflection. First, there are issues in dispute. Some scholars, even sympathetic ones, have sought to demonstrate that poverty and poor health are not inextricably linked.[137] But the problem will not go away. As Horton and Leslie argue:

> Ill-health is probably the greatest single cause of human suffering. . . . It is doubtful if any other single circumstance produces so much poverty and dependency, so much family disruption, or so much economic inefficiency as illness . . .[138]

There are countless other indicators, including infant and maternal morbidity, premature deaths, and lost workdays. For example, due to inadequate or nonexistent prenatal care, black children are far more likely than white children to be born premature. And infants born prematurely are 16 times more likely to die during the neonatal period (the first 28 days of life) and 10 times more likely to be retarded.[139] More data could be recited; books and articles abound, and are sent to congressmen and senators every day. There are analytic debating points: does poverty "cause" ill-health or are the two simply found together with more than average frequency, and so on.

But the point is basic. By almost any measure, the poor are sicker than the nonpoor, and medicine does not cure them, even though the poorest see physicians as often as the more affluent. The reason is that it is not medicine alone that the poor need. Health is not the product of the multiplication of services and people; it is rather a function of a health-producing environment and individual energy. The poor have neither. Two of the greatest insults that poverty inflicts are the narrowness of options and vitiation of energy. The debate about access to medical care misses a more fundamental point. The poor need medical care, but only to achieve a threshold condition, a state that can make other things possible.

Unless medicine is reconceived, the poor may continue to

receive care but be sicker in the year 2000. Of all the factors that might be mitigated, and thus cause more rather than less health over the next few decades, poverty is the least likely candidate. This society has chosen to shatter the lives of the poor and nourish the rich. That choice is unlikely to be reversed voluntarily.

THE DIVERGENCE OF
MEDICINE AND SOCIETY

Medicine and society are diverging. As we saw in Chapter 3, an increase in transnational activity, on both public and private levels, will result in health problems that transcend national boundaries at a time when all nations, including the United States, are elaborating and expanding their own medical care systems to the exclusion of the development of a world health care system. In this chapter, we have seen that, by the year 2000:

1. Increases in complexity, stress, the size of organizations, and the persistence of work-related stress will present society with new and aggravated health problems. Thus, while certain technological improvements such as the rapid development of the computer offer opportunities to improve medical care, unforeseen health care problems may arise in the future.

2. Leaving aside emerging health problems, over the next 30 years life is likely to be more stressful, faster, and more frenetic than it is now. The diseases of civilization, such as heart disease, vascular disorders, and cancer, will exact an even higher toll because medicine is oriented toward their cure, not their prevention.

3. The population will be older. Although the health care system will fail to "cure" old age, it will nevertheless continue to lavish resources on the elderly.

4. The number of accidental deaths and injuries will continue to rise (even if in step with population growth), yet medicine engages the problem only after the fact, and poorly when it does.

5. There is solid evidence that environmental degradation damages health and is increasing in magnitude. But medicine is designed only to repair human machinery at a time when the theoretical and empirical evidence is that health is substantially more determined by social and environmental factors.

6. The degree of mental and emotional disorder may be increasing. Levels of mental and emotional disorder may be exacerbated in the future by psychological pressures on the aged as a result of expanded longevity and expulsion from the job market. But there is little evidence that mental health services have a measurable impact on the incidence of mental illness. Under such circumstances, not only might mental and emotional disorders increase, their debilitating impact on society is unlikely to be affected by the provision of services. Once again social causes deserve more attention.

7. Biomedical breakthroughs promise to improve the tools of the medical care system to treat certain conditions, mostly acute in nature. At the same time, such technological innovations have made and will make it possible for the system to expand the present style of treatment almost infinitely. The result has been and will be high costs and more concentration on acute conditions by increasingly specialized practitioners.

8. Poverty will not be "cured."

9. Professionalism in medicine, which heavily influences its reductionist drift and depersonalizes medical care interactions, is incompatible with the values of a growing number of persons. One result is that the mode of administration of medical care, and even its logos, will be increasingly dissonant with emerging human values and needs.

10. Finally, because of the lock on services by service

bureaucracies, the provision of medical care will become more political because of the pursuit of internal objectives by service bureaucracies to the derogation of consumer rights and interests.

A new medicine is needed. The old medicine has reached its limits; it can no longer cure more than harm.

5

The Climate for Medicine

The real revolution in medicine, like all real revolutions, will
go on at the level of conceptions.
                        Andrew Weil, *The Natural Mind*

We have the medicine we deserve. We freely choose to live
the way we do. We choose to live recklessly, to abuse our
bodies with what we consume, to expose ourselves to environmental insults, to rush frantically from place to place,
and to sit on our spreading bottoms and watch paid professionals exercise for us. Because this is the way most of us live
we need a medicine that repairs us when our systems break
down. This is essentially what modern medicine tries to do.
And it is something that medicine generally does well. But
the climate for a "reparative" medicine is changing. The
assaults on our health are different now, even though our
life styles compel medicine to stay where it is. Will we
change; will medicine change?

Thus far I have tried to demonstrate three propositions.
First, medical care has less impact on health than is generally
assumed. Second, medical care has less impact on health
than have social and environmental factors. And third, given
the way in which society is evolving and the evolutionary
imperatives of the medical care system, medical care in the
future will have even less impact on health than it has now.

Most of my argument has been supported by findings
drawn from conventional research. But the argument thus

far has taken medical care on its own terms—measuring it by what it tries to do. There are other powerful, even profound, reasons why the end of medicine is near, however. The societal web in which medicine is a thick strand is unraveling. Changes now occurring in society will fuel the dissolution of the medical care system and, more importantly, lead to a redefinition of health.

The times must be ripe for any change. There must be an accumulation of insight, criticism, consciousness, and political acumen at one end of a teeter-totter so that the medicine of today, at the other end, can be tipped. Sudden changes can occur—intellectual history reveals the suddenness of some transformations. Sufficient weight is now accumulating; a shift in social and political vision is coming. Modern medicine will then appear as it is—an anachronism.

AN EMERGING ZEITGEIST

There is a growing, almost palpable sense that our culture is at an epoch break, that a major transformation to something new and different and possibly better lies ahead. The "transformation," to use George Leonard's word,[1] is based in a sharp alteration in our image of reality.

Leonard suggests that the shifts in Western scientific thought outlined in Thomas Kuhn's *The Structure of Scientific Revolutions*[2] yield clues to what is occurring. Kuhn uses the term "paradigm." By this he means the assumptions, premises, and glue that hold together a prevailing interpretation of reality. Paradigms are rigid, even religious. Even up to the point where the paradigm breaks down, phenomena must either fit or be shoved into the paradigm as they are discovered. But new paradigms can emerge from the old when the explanatory power of the old is exhausted. Leonard describes some of the boundary conditions for change:

The new paradigm appears and prevails only if the old one is in a state of crisis, only when the older mode of investigation seems to be producing a series of anomalies and is running into increasing difficulties with certain key questions of the times.[3]

He then argues that the threshold of a major societal transformation has been reached—a transformation manifesting a reverence for life and joy, rather than despair in living, and ushering in an era of cooperation and communality to replace the divisiveness and brutishness that characterize our lives today.

Leonard is the most animated and expressive millenarian at work. But for all of his effusiveness, his vision lacks the analytic rigor necessary to convert the hardhearted. Jonas Salk supplies some rigor in *The Survival of the Wisest.*[4] However, he is not without his own brand of "mysticism."

> a new body of conscious individuals exists expressing its desire for a better life for Man as a species and as individuals, eager to devote themselves to this end. Such groups, when they are able to coalesce through an understanding of their relatedness to one another and to the natural processes involved in "Nature's game" of survival and evolution, will find strength and courage in sensing themselves as a part of the Cosmos and as being involved in a game that is in accord with Nature and not anti-natural. These groups will initiate movements, which in turn will be manifest in their effect not only upon the species and the planet but upon individual lives. Their benefit is likely to be expressed in a greater satisfaction and fulfillment in life.[5]

Like other contributors to the recent literature, Salk postulates the necessity of a new consciousness. His book is a biological counterpart to a dialogue begun by ecologists such as Barry Commoner and Garrett Hardin, quantitative scientists such as Meadows and the members of the Club of Rome, and social philosophers such as Ivan Illich and George Leonard. But Salk's work is unique because, of those who have argued that growth must be limited, only he has also offered an argument that man is equal to the task.

Jonas Salk is a highly trained and sophisticated life scientist. Hence, it is from the world of biological science that his images evolve. His argument is simple. In nature all animals, including human beings, survive on the basis of principles of natural selection. Nature "chooses" from a "blooming profusion" of choices those life forms with survival value. The theory is clean, neat, and mechanistic. One species of moth survives because a random mutation in the coloration of its wings happily blends into the field of flora in which it lives; another is decimated by predators because its wing coloration contrasts rather than merges with the backdrop.

This is essentially, so the theory goes, how human life evolved. And this is where Salk starts to analogize. His reasoning runs something like this: If there are unmistakable signs of decay in our culture—the population explosion (upon which he relies heavily), environmental degradation, wide-ranging mental instability, endless war and conflict—then for that culture to survive, it must evolve. In short, according to Salk, it must reestablish a harmonious relationship with its surroundings. But this can only take place through natural selection; nature will judge us for our survival value. Salk argues that we must therefore create and then share ideas that have survival value. The rubric Salk attaches to this process is "metabiology." If the biological refers to the stuff and substance of life, then the metabiological consists of sociocultural ideas, myths, and consciousness, which, as in the case of corporeal life, are selected for their value in the preservation of the species.

What is novel about Salk's thinking is that it can now be made public by such a distinguished scientist and scholar. But his argument for the need for a new consciousness is far from fresh. The same point has been made by many, from Thoreau to Gandhi to Maslow. Those who argue that hu-

manity has reached an epoch break, a point of transition to a
new era and a new humanity, are not lonely voices in the
wilderness but part of a growing chorus. There are fundamentally two arguments. The first, which foresees the end of
civilization, the dissolution of culture, is well represented by
Lewis Mumford in *The Myth of the Machine,* by William Irwin
Thompson in *At the Edge of History* and *Passages About Earth,*
and by George Leonard. Some of these commentators, such
as Leonard, have gone on to the second argument—that a
new epoch is emerging, or at least that we are on its
threshold. It has become less and less easy to dismiss these
voices as millenarian, rustic, nonscientific, or even crazy.

A rich diversity of views characterize the debate. But there
are a few fundamental principles:

1.   As a civilization we are spent. Sociocultural innovation
is impoverished, and economic and political structures are
variations on a common and empty theme. Revolutions and
revolts, each chasing on the heels of its predecessor, disappear one into another in a dreary uniformity—the op-
pressed become the oppressors, and so on. In *The Struggle
Against History,* Ronald Segal, a socialist critic and writer,
recognizes this when he says of the two dominant political
and economic systems: "While the two . . . competitively
pursue the development of their material technology,
neither seems capable of developing ideas or institutions to
reorganize society on more creative moral lines."[6]

2.   Our technology has brought us to ruin. We are
poisoning our environment beyond repair. Remedial programs utilizing still more technology are ultimately self-
defeating. There are flaws inherent in technological
problem-solving. Moreover, there may be fixed and immutable limits to growth, even though we do not know when we
shall reach them. Robert Theobald puts it this way in *Habit
and Habitat:*

All other species work within the existing habitat. Their success or failure depends upon their ability to adapt to the conditions in which they find themselves. Their survival depends upon a complex, interrelated ecosystem of which they form a small part and over which they have very limited control. . . .

Man alone has tried to deny his relationship to the total ecosystem of which he forms part by continuously ignoring and cutting off feedback which he finds undesirable. He has developed the habit of seeing his habitat as totally flexible according to his own wishes and desires.[7]

3.   Our science is far more "relative" than we have assumed. Neither its contents nor its methods are absolute. Prevailing paradigms springing from materialistic and mechanistic bases are blurring at the edges. Although the behavioral sciences continue to rely largely on traditional interpretations, the physical sciences are striding into mysticism. Hence, to assume that a linear development of current scientific knowledge will subsume the usable knowledge of the future is to fall into what Richard H. Bube, a professor of material sciences and electrical engineering at Stanford University, has labeled "one of the most pernicious falsehoods ever to be almost universally accepted."

4.   When taken together, the similar strands woven through existing mythic, religious, and scientific accounts suggest a "lost" historical record. These provocative strands are found in the records of the Sumerian culture and the ancient cultures of Central America, particularly Mexico. The "myth" of Atlantis provides another example.

5.   We are all familiar to one degree or another with the recrudescence of the occult. N. Freedland traced the revival in *The Occult Explosion*,[8] and Colin Wilson rendered its historical sweep in *The Occult*.[9] Moreover, new religious movements are springing up. Edgar Cayce has been more widely read than nearly any other author in recent years. J. R. R. Tolkien's "Ring" trilogy is in its fiftieth printing.[10] These

movements may be mere crescendos, but they may also augur a more durable cultural transformation.

6. Our perceptions of reality may be incorrect, or at least greatly distorted. The anthropological lore of Carlos Castaneda is perhaps the best single statement.[11] Like Don Juan's teachings presented by Castaneda, the world view of the Hopi and some Eastern beliefs are consistent in their fusion of mind and body, and of matter, energy, and consciousness, even though those terms have been used unrigorously. Sartre touches on this in his tetralogy, *The Roads to Freedom*,[12] when he depicts Mathieu's wonderment at the pulsing life of a tree. George Leonard in *The Transformation* picks up the theme this way:

> For a brief moment I experienced the tree's being, then I am thrust back firmly to my separate existence, capable of seeing the tree at a distance, touching it, cutting it down, analyzing it. I have been given names for each of its constituent parts, terms for its processes, and ways for relating it with the other elements of the biosphere. But I have been made incapable of entering its being and sharing its life. . . .
>
> But something is wrong with this mode of perceiving and being, even in strictly scientific terms. The physicists have taught me that the tree, so substantial and impenetrable, actually is mostly "empty space"; if we conceive the subatomic elements of which it is made as particles. . . . Therefore, the tree appears impenetrable to my physical body, a handy correspondence. Its opacity, however, is operational, not ultimate. Physics and mathematics have provided us a respectable way of acknowledging what primitive peoples have always known: The tree is not really solid. There is room in it for spirits.[13]

7. Related to the issue of reality is the anthropocentricism of our science, which persists in classifying homo sapiens as a wholly independent variable in the cosmos. Much of the cosmic literature is sensationalized; Hal Lindsey's *The Late, Great Planet Earth* is an example.[14] But as William Irwin Thompson has said:

something is carrying on an extended communication through the opening and closing of our Epoch, with the information cells of our civilization. "Jesus people" would say it is Christ preparing for his Second Coming; pagans would say it is the return of the gods in their flying saucers; technologists would say . . . that it is not to the heavens that we should look for an explanation, but to earth: they themselves are the new gods who are ending the trivial culture of homo sapiens. . .[15]

8.   Many argue that the dominant culture of consumption and competition must yield to an emergent culture characterized by self-restraint, cooperation, and communality. These views have not found their way into politics, but they may form the foundation for the future social experimentation.

9.   In ways that are not entirely clear, there are signs of an evolving "consciousness" among an increasing, largely youthful, but still small number of people. This evolution both derives from and animates the other principles of change.

A New "Naturalism."   A host of observers, including Charles Reich, Jonas Salk, Theodore Roszak, George Leonard, and Kenneth Kenniston, perceive the growth of a new counterculture. There is general agreement that there is a movement to build a better, more humane society, but observers disagree on the causes, breadth, and specific aims of the movement. In an article in *Saturday Review*, "The New Naturalism," Daniel Yankelovich argues that the new naturalism means, among other things:

> To push the Darwinian version of nature as "survival of the fittest" into the background, and to emphasize instead the interdependence of all things and species in nature;
> To place sensory experience ahead of conceptual knowledge;
> To live physically close to nature, in the open, off the land;

To live in groups (tribes, communes) rather than in such "artificial" social units as the nuclear family;

To de-emphasize aspects of nature illumined by science; instead, to celebrate all the unknown, the mystical, and the mysterious elements of nature;

To stress cooperation rather than competition;

To devalue detachment, objectivity, and noninvolvement as methods for finding truth; to arrive at truth, instead, by direct experience, participation and involvement;

To reject mastery over nature;

To emphasize the community rather than the individual; and

To preserve the environment at the expense of economic growth and technology.[16]

The implications of this change are difficult to draw. But if the movement gains momentum over the next three decades, new values will be established upon which future decisions must be based. One outcome may be further discrediting of the growth principle. If so, some of the problems associated with growth, such as pollution, resource depletion, and the spread of concrete might be checked.[17]

The projected increased age of the population is also pertinent. If it is true that attitudes engendered in youth survive into old age, many of those who govern at the end of this century will have been acculturated differently from those who govern today. Although the countercultural revolution may turn out to be ephemeral, it is still likely to have some effect on political and social change over the next 30 years.

There are three related implications for medicine. First, the idea of community implies increased local control. The medical care system has been slowly integrating and enlarging. With that integration has come a steady inflation of the role of the federal government. The passage of a national health insurance plan will swell the federal role even more. But at the same time, some communities may seek to assume more, not less, of the obligation to provide their care. In addition, consumer demands for more personalized care are likely to increase; ironically at a time when manpower shortages and the institutionalization in the medical care system frustrates this demand.

Second, we may see a return to folk medicine. It is doubtful that this will be widespread, but communities may try to treat "their own" using indigenous folk practices. The women's movement, for one, has encouraged self-care programs. The demise of folk medicine was associated with the disintegration of viable insular communities.[18] With the recrudescence of community, new folk practices, possibly more scientifically based, may evolve.[19]

The final implication may be the most significant. Professionalism is incompatible with the idea of community and the egalitarianism that accompanies it. But professionalism in the sense of autonomy, to use Eliot Freidson's conceptualization, is the cornerstone of the medical care system. A successful attack on it may shake the edifice.[20] If the attack on professional prerogatives by new naturalists is coupled with a rational systemic critique, the trend to a different medicine may be accelerated.

Higher Consciousness. In *The Natural Mind,*[21] Andrew Weil draws a distinction between "straight," or conventional thinking, and "stoned" thinking. Straight thinking is characterized as:

- a tendency to know things through the intellect rather than through some faculty of mind;
- a tendency to be attached to the senses and through them to external reality;
- a tendency to pay attention to outward forms rather than to inner contents and thus to lapse into materialism;

- a tendency to perceive differences rather than similarities among phenomena;
- a tendency toward negative thinking, pessimism, and despair.

The use of insecticides exemplifies straight thinking, according to Weil. Straight thinking assumes that nature is hostile and can be managed by direct application of force. Weil continues:

> As vigorous selective agents, insecticides in our world play a significant role in the evolutionary development of all insect species. They neatly weed out the susceptible number of families concentrating in insect gene pools all over the world the genetic factors that confer resistance to these chemicals.[22]

The continued use of insecticides creates new, resistant strains of insects through natural selection. New and more effective insecticides are then needed and so on—an infinite regress.

Weil then distinguishes straight thinking from "stoned" thinking:

- a reliance on intuition as well as intellection;
- an acceptance of the ambivalent nature of things;
- an experience of infinity and its positive aspects.

The autonomic nervous system, which is supposed to trigger the involuntary muscles such as the heart, illustrates stoned thinking. Under prevailing biomedical concepts, the autonomic nervous system is not "connected" to consciousness. Weil disagrees. He alludes to hypnotic suggestion. If told that his or her skin has been touched by hot metal, a subject in full trance will blister as if burned when touched by a finger. Weil concludes that there "must be a channel between mind and body [that] is wide open whenever we are in an altered state of consciousness."[23] Biofeedback research supports Weil's argument.[24]

States of consciousness, beyond those generally experienced, are a theme in many contemporary works.[25] Many commentators feel there are means to elevate human consciousness to a higher plane. In *The Master Game*,[26] one of the many books and articles on the subject, Robert S. De-Ropp argues that because human beings have evolved with a large brain, they should be capable of far greater powers than they have demonstrated. DeRopp feels that, "because [man] does not know how to use this powerful machine, it tends to operate in ways not beneficial to its possessor, to generate a host of illusions among which he wanders . . . frightened and confused, a prey to terrors that he himself has created."[27] The argument is far from new. William James made the same point in *The Varieties of Religious Experience* in 1929:

> One conclusion forced upon my mind at that time, and my impression of its truth has ever since remained unshaken. It is that our normal waking consciousness, rational consciousness as we call it, is but one special type of consciousness, whilst all about it, parted from it by the filmiest of screens, there lie potential forms of consciousness entirely different. We may go through life without suspecting their existence, but apply the requisite stimulus, and at a touch they are there in all their completeness. . . . No account of the universe in its totality can be final which leaves these other forms of consciousness quite disregarded.[28]

There are many implications for medical care. If human beings are capable of higher states of consciousness, it may be possible for individuals to assume more responsibility for self-care than is now the case (even among those who have not succumbed to professional coercions). There will also be a larger role for natural healers. The literature, flanked by a wealth of anecdotal accounts, is full of descriptions of natural healings.[29]

It is possible that healing in the future will be based upon a more complete understanding of the role of consciousness. The mechanistic approach to health and well-being that characterizes modern medicine is inconsistent with concepts of higher consciousness. The more that is discovered about human potential and the powers of an evolved consciousness, the less sense the prevailing medical paradigm makes. We may be at the limits of allopathic medicine to treat and reduce disease; new approaches are needed, new ways to heal and be healed. Some diseases may result from imbalances in consciousness that can only be treated through its alteration. It may then be possible to achieve improvements in health through expanding consciousness.[30]

Medicine is a part of the culture in which it is practiced. If transformations take place that alter the beliefs and attitudes underlying our culture, medicine will inevitably be affected.

MEDICINE, SOCIETY, AND CULTURE

Modern medicine arose in a hospital environment. But the climate for a medicine that only cures is chilling.

Ecology.   Barry Commoner, in *The Closing Circle,*[31] postulates four laws of ecology: "(1) everything is connected to everything else; (2) everything must go somewhere; (3) nature knows best; and (4) there is no such thing as a free lunch." In his discussion, Commoner condemns the scientific community in pertinent terms:

> Few of us in the scientific community are well prepared to deal with this degree of complexity. We have been trained by modern science to think about events that are vastly more simple—how one particle bounces off another, or how Molecule A reacts with Molecule B. Confronted by a situation as complex as the environment and its vast array of living

inhabitants, we are likely—some more than others—to attempt to reduce it in our minds to a set of separate, simple events, in the hope that their sum will somehow picture the whole. The existence of the environmental crisis warns us that this is an illusory hope. For some time now, biologists have studied isolated animals and plants, and biochemists have studied molecules isolated in test tubes, accumulating the vast, detailed literature of modern biological science. Yet these separate data have yielded no sums that explain the ecology of a lake, for instance, and its vulnerability.[32]

The earth on which we live—the ecosphere—is where health takes place. It is where we are well or not well. This is not a simple-minded nostrum, for upon reflection it is clear that unless ill health is the product of evil spirits, the causes of disease can be found in the ecosphere and in man's manipulation of its elements. It follows that prevention and even treatment of disease lies in fostering conditions that are conducive to health. As our ecological knowledge grows, the impoverishment of our approach to health will become increasingly evident. This approach to health is not novel (I discuss some of its roots later), but it has not been cogently expressed as a guide for action.

Systems. In the preface to *Habit and Habitat,* Robert Theobald distinguishes man's relationship to his habitat from that of other species:

> Man is unique. This statement has been made so often—and so incorrectly—that we have lost sight of the few areas where it is profoundly true. In particular, we fail to remember that man is the only species which had developed the means to force his habitat into patterns which he desires. He has used ever-greater power to enable him to do what he wants to do and prevent those patterns which he finds undesirable.[33]

Theobald then develops the thesis that the solution to the environmental crisis depends upon a change in the means by which we reach decisions. The change Theobald has in mind is from a linear hierarchic approach to decision-making to what he refers to as a "sapiential" view, one that relies on the wisdom and knowledge of the individual free of rigid institutional constraints. He stops short of arguing for a fundamental change in consciousness, but not too short; changing decision-making requires changes in the mental and emotional equipment we bring to the problem. Theobald's plea is simple: We must develop the capacity to approach our world and its problems systemically through the use of sapiential analysis. These are modes of analysis that do not tie individuals up in institutions that filter information for their own purposes. Sapiential analysis compels us to be sensitive to the feedback we get from the subjects affected by our initiatives, and, crucially, to make adjustments in the mixture of inputs we bring to bear upon those subjects.

Our technology has made it possible to massively rearrange our environment to suit our needs. We have raped the earth in order to tame it. We have eliminated or altered what we found either distasteful or inconvenient. If a river was not straight, we straightened it. If a forest made it difficult to build our homes or facilitate our commerce, we removed it. Since we found it more convenient to dump our waste products on the land and in the lakes and oceans than to recycle it, we did so.

This is what modern medicine does as well—it removes problems. It fixes on undesirable symptoms and tries to eliminate them rather than addressing their causes. But the feedback we are getting from the spaceship in which we live—befouled air, fetid water, human flotsam, and noise—is forcing us to calibrate exploitation of our environment with its limitations. We are slowly being forced to respect our environment. The methodology by which we will do so is systemic in nature. We must approach the problem of health in the same terms.

We are not getting healthier any more, as we did for many

centuries. This may be because our medicine has not respected the interconnectedness of the human organism and its environment. We have not fully understood the extent to which our health is dependent on our overall environment. When public health measures succeeded in cleansing water and disposing of waste, society forgot the lessons we learned from those programs. We succumbed to conceptual cowardice and miscomprehended the systemic nature of our existence. We then embarked on the pursuit of health by assuming we could deal with the human organism in isolation from its society and its environment. But as Kenneth Boulding has said:

> We must get the idea across that society is a great pond, and just as in a fish pond (if it's unpolluted) frogs, vegetation and chemicals all interact to form a reasonably stable equilibrium of populations, so in society we have rough equilibrium at any one moment of interacting populations of criminals, police, automobiles, schools, churches, supermarkets, nations, armies, corporations, laws, universities and ideas.[34]

Values. Today science is under attack because it has lusted after means and been blind to ends. Science will survive the attack because it will adjust and because we cannot do without it. But it will be forced to retrench, and in doing so will be compelled to enter human values into its equations. It will be forced to subject the ends it pursues to the assent of those who are affected.

Medicine is part of the scientific community. This accounts for its successes and for some of the critique lodged against it as well. Medicine, along with the other sciences, has elaborated its means and forgotten its ends. If health had been the objective we would be healthier. But health has not been the objective. The objective has been technique. Jacques Ellul described this dichotomy in *The Technological Society*[35] when he pointed out that elaboration of technique and man's inability to control the technology he has created is due to our failure to understand how to change the underlying set of assumptions from which we work. This is true of medicine as well.

We generally assume that technology is, or at least can be, value-free. But technology is not value-free. In Guatemala, the tourist who takes a photograph of a native has "captured" the soul of his subject. At least that is what some natives believe. The subject returns to his hut, desists from further human interaction, and refuses to eat and care for himself. He may die shortly thereafter. To the technocrat this episode is indubitable evidence of primitive foolishness and stupidity. The camera, he asserts, is merely a device for passively recording physical phenomena and can in no way harm the subject. While this view may assuage any guilt the tourist may have, it is of little solace to the native. It is, rather, an arrogance borne out of benign assumptions about tools and technology that leads the technocrat to his interpretation. But the fact remains that since the camera can *cause* the native's death, it can hardly, under these circumstances, be considered value-free. All technology carries the potential for human harm. The fact that the threat is "merely" in the eyes of the beholder is not an argument to the contrary.

Value judgments are common features of medical practice. When many of us were born, typically, our mothers were anesthetized, and our fathers condemned to dingy, magazine littered waiting rooms. We were born blue and silent. Shortly after that, we and our mothers were confined to quarters for roughly five days. Our fathers were allowed to visit a few hours a day, sharing their time with friends and relatives who crowded in to applaud the result. Today in some hospitals mothers and fathers are both in the delivery room participating in the birth of a writhing pink infant who rips the air with sound as soon as its chest cavity is free. The health of the parties to this scenario—the baby, the mother, and the father—is not adversely affected by the change in medical practice. The practice of medicine is heavily laden with value judgments. There is nothing in the physician's technical armamentarium that dictates one scenario over another. The presence or absence of a father, and the drugging of the mother or her sentiency are societal values that the physician mirrors in his practice.

A sense of the values implicit in medicine is rare among practitioners. In part this is due to the insularity health practitioners have bred for themselves. At the core of medicine is the concept of autonomy, which is a function of specialized knowledge and methods. The training of a physician is the progressive enshrinement of specialized information. At the end of the educational process, licensing serves as the final rites of passage.

But training and initiation involve more than that. The medical student is made to feel quite different from other students. The student-would-be-professional is inculcated with the quaint notion that the knowledge he or she gains can be transformed into a service which is, by that fact, salable for a price. This is distinguishable from the view of the nonprofessional. For example, the sociologist seldom views his or her knowledge as dangerous in the hands of a nonsociologist, nor readily convertible into a service that can be rendered for a price.

An unarticulated premise of medical training is that the knowledge imparted in the process is unique and nonfungible; in short, a commodity for market exchange. As such, a physician's knowledge is neither an end in itself nor a contributor to the fund of human knowledge; it is, rather, synonymous with technique, because it is useful only when applied to a problem. It has its own technological imperative as well, which is largely the same as that of other technology in that its existence compels its use, but somewhat different in that its use is strictly limited to those who are its purveyors.

This apotheosis of technique has shorn medicine of a sense of values and stripped us of our capacity to take responsibility for our own health.

Reality. Our science and our religion tell us what is real. But of course there are "unreal" things. In *The Teachings of Don Juan: A Yaqui Way of Knowledge,* Carlos Castaneda describes the "unreal" when he recounts his first "flying" experience:

> Don Juan kept staring at me. I took a step toward him. My legs were rubbery and long, extremely long. I took another step. My knee joints felt springy, like a vault pole; they shook and vibrated and contracted elastically. I moved forward. The motion of my body was slow and shaky; it was more like a tremor forward and up. I looked down and saw don Juan sitting below me, way below me. The momentum carried me forward one more step, which was even more elastic and longer than the preceding one. And from there I soared. I remember coming down once; then I pushed up with both feet, sprang backward, and glided on my back. I saw the dark sky above me, and the clouds going by me. I jerked my body so I could look down. I saw the dark mass of the mountains. My speed was extraordinary. My arms were fixed, folded against my sides. . . .
>
> The same day, Friday, July 5, late in the afternoon, don Juan asked me to narrate the details of my experience. As carefully as I could, I related the whole episode. . . . Finally, before I left that evening, I had to ask him, "Did I really fly, don Juan?"
>
> "That is what you told me. Didn't you?"
>
> "I know, don Juan. I mean, did my body fly? Did I take off like a bird?"
>
> "You always ask me questions I cannot answer. You flew . . . [T]he trouble with you is that you understand things in only one way. You don't think a man flies; and yet a brujo can move a thousand miles in one second to see what is going on. He can deliver a blow to his enemies long distances away. So, does he or doesn't he fly?"

"You see, don Juan, you and I are differently oriented. Suppose, for the sake of argument, one of my fellow students had been here with me when I took the devil's weed. Would he have been able to see me flying?"

"There you go again with your questions about what would happen if. . . It is useless to talk that way. If your friend, or anybody else, takes the second portion of the weed all he can do is fly. Now, if he had simply watched you, he might have seen you flying, or he might not. That depends on the man."

"But what I mean, don Juan, is that if you and I look at a bird and see it fly, we agree that it is flying. But if two of my friends had seen me flying as I did last night, would they have agreed that I was flying?"

"Well, they might have. You agree that birds fly because you have seen them flying. Flying is a common thing with birds. But you will not agree on other things birds do, because you have never seen birds do them. If your friends knew about men flying with the devil's weed, then they would agree."

"Let's put it another way, don Juan. What I meant to say is that if I had tied myself to a rock with a heavy chain, I would have flown just the same, because my body had nothing to do with my flying."

Don Juan looked at me incredulously. "If you tie yourself to a rock," he said, "I'm afraid you will have to fly holding the rock with its heavy chain."[36]

Slowly but steadily we are discovering the flimsiness of our reality. Interest in the unconscious, the unknown, and the occult is reawakening, however long vitiated by our assumption that the mind consisted only of the intellect. The bifurcation of mind and body, and our belief that the unconscious mind is the home of the chaotic and the irrational are characteristics of this technological era. Yet breakthroughs occur. Higher consciousness is possible—different and more penetrating visions of reality are possible. Some are drug-induced, but the most lucid are not. Nevertheless, the paradigms of the past are firmly entrenched. To Theodore Roszak, in *Where the Wasteland Ends*,[37] the prevailing paradigm rests on a "myth of objective consciousness." For

Roszak the myth is not necessarily false, but rather an idiom of explanation which filters out phenomena that do not fit. This results in "reductionism," which Roszak sees as the desire to "reduce all things to terms that objective consciousness might master."

This reliance on material reality and its accompanying reduction of subject matter to manageable, quantifiable, and discrete parts characterizes medicine. Medicine focuses on the smallest bits of material reality—symptoms—and ignores a buzzing profusion of phenomena which may be related to health.

In *The Natural Mind,* Andrew Weil characterizes medicine's preoccupation with material reality this way:

> Modern allopathic medicine is essentially materialistic. For example, the widely accepted germ theory of disease—a cornerstone of allopathic theory—states that certain microscopic entities (bacteria and viruses are the most important) whose appearance in space and time correlates well with other physical manifestations of illness are causative of illness.[38]

In contrast, Weil stresses the importance of the "unconscious" in achieving health. Whether Weil is right in his assumptions about health, an issue to which I return, his diagnosis of modern medicine's perceptions of reality is accurate. But perceptions of reality can change. As society shifts from its mechanistic and materialistic bases, it will strip medicine of its premises.

Paranormal Phenomena. In 1909, when Freud and Jung were in the spring of their collaboration, Jung engaged Freud in a discussion of extrasensory perception. Jung recounts one of their talks:

> While Freud was going on this way, I had a curious sensation. It was as if my diaphragm was made of iron and was becoming

red hot—a glowing vault. At that moment there was such a loud report in the bookcase which stood right next to us that we both started up in alarm fearing the thing was going to topple over us. I said to Freud: "There, that is an example of a so-called catalytic exteriorization phenomenon."

"Oh, come!" "That is sheer bosh."

"It is not," I replied. "You are mistaken Herr Professor. But to prove my point I now predict that in a moment there will be another loud report." Sure enough, no sooner had I said the words than detonation went off in the bookcase.[39]

Other incidents of exteriorization or psychokinesis are reported by Ostrander and Schroeder in *Psychic Discoveries Behind the Iron Curtain*.[40] In their book they narrate episodes about Nelya Mikhailova, one of the persons they observed in the Soviet Union. Among other things, Nelya was apparently able to move objects around on a table without touching them. When doing so, her pulse rate escalated rapidly to nearly 200 beats per minute; and she often lost three to six pounds when she worked. Leaving aside the obvious implications for weight control, her performance is remarkable. So remarkable that some skeptics have pointed out that Nelya was given a jail sentence in 1964 for some unspecified crime. Ostrander and Schroeder claim it was for some unrelated petty offense, but the skeptics argue that it was for chicanery.

Supporters, including Koestler, point out that Nelya is a high-spirited woman who is often a prankster in her work—a little like the brain surgeon who propositions the scrub nurse while gingerly separating brain tissues. But some critics have been unsparing, and an author of Koestler's caliber should not uncritically accept secondhand accounts. In fairness, the weight of the evidence is on Koestler's side.

There have been enough events like those reported by Ostrander and Schroeder, many verified by dubious scholars, to conclude that paranormal events do occur. In *The*

Roots of Coincidence,[41] Koestler tries to introduce "respectability" to the parapsychological field.[42] An example of research recited by Koestler is a study conducted by scientists at the University of Hawaii. The following is an extract of their project report:

> To make a fresh start (and perhaps to confuse the opposition) they [MacBain and his group] have abandoned the term ESP, with its rather negative connotations, and coined the new term quasi-sensory communications, or QSC for short. They also formulated a simple basic hypothesis: "If one individual has access to information not available to another, then under certain circumstances and with known sensory channels rigidly controlled, the second individual can demonstrate knowledge of this information at a higher level than that compatible with the alternative explanation of chance guessing." And then they set out to test it—with most intriguing results.
>
> For their subjects they used 22 volunteer psychology students, who operated in pairs. . . The information to be communicated consisted of a set of 23 concepts which seemed likely to evoke a wide range of emotional reactions, and which could be symbolized by simple line drawings (including, for example, home, sleep, sorrow, sunshine, and the Pill). Each pair of students used just five of these concepts. The sender in each pair sat at a row of five display panels, one of which was illuminated for 25 seconds. The receiver faced a similar row of the five symbols, all illuminated, with a button below each. He used the appropriate button to signal the concept he thought had been "transmitted" by the sender. The sender had to concentrate on the illuminated symbol for 25 seconds, and then relax for 5 seconds while the receiver made a choice. Receiver and sender were in separate rooms over 30 feet apart. . . .
>
> The actual results . . . were significantly different from . . . random distribution. . . . This means that chance guessing alone is not enough to explain the results. . .[43]

Koestler also recounts an experiment conducted by W. Gray Walter, a leading neurophysiologist in England. Walter's experimental approach can be described this way. Electrodes are attached to the scalp over the subject's frontal

cortex to transmit electrical brain activities through an
amplifier to a machine. In front of the subject there is a
button which, if pressed, causes an "interesting scene" to
appear on a television screen. About one second before the
subject presses the button an electrical charge occurs in a
large area of the subject's cortex. This is referred to as the
"readiness wave." The circuits of the apparatus can also be
adjusted so that the readiness wave can trigger a switch and
make the TV scene appear a fraction of a second before the
subject actually presses the button.

Intelligent subjects soon realize that what they "intend"
"produces" the expected result before they have actually
moved a finger. Soon they cease to press the button; the
pictures appear when they want them. To sustain the effect,
it is essential that subjects "want" the event to occur, and
concentrate on it occurring. When subjects' attention wanders, as for example with a monotonous presentation, or if
they concentrate on concentration, they receive no pictures.
Autostart can be combined with autostop so that subjects can
generate a picture by willing its appearance on the TV
screen, and then can erase it as soon as they have completed their review.[44]

There are many other examples of paranormal phenomena. A number of them are chronicled by Andrija Puharich,
a physician who has worked extensively with psychics and
healers. Puharich reports much of his research in his book,
Beyond Telepathy.[45] But far more startling is his account of his
experiences and research with Uri Geller, a young Israeli, in
his book *Uri*.[46] Geller's feats have been widely reported.[47]
But Puharich adds rich details. Of particular interest are the
findings of the Stanford Research Institute (SRI) reported in
Nature.[48] At Puharich's urging, SRI, the largest private
nonprofit research center in the United States, examined
Geller in an attempt to verify his paranormal skills. Unfortunately, the material released thus far by SRI is limited to
telepathy and clairvoyance.[49] In each case, however, the re-

ports are confirmatory and extraordinary, although some have questioned the research methods. Geller was able to identify which box contained a metal airplane at odds of one million to one. He also reproduced instantaneously and with great accuracy drawings done by others miles away.

In *Uri*, Puharich describes activities not yet reported by SRI. These include psychokinesis—bending metal objects, moving objects, stopping and starting watches—and materialization and dematerialization. This is strange stuff. But it is enjoying more acceptance than ever, in part because physics itself, the most sublime of the sciences, is moving in strange directions.

Koestler stresses the convergence of theoretical physics and parapsychological phenomenon. In a chapter entitled "The Perversity of Physics," he assesses the emerging body of theory and its trajectory into the mysterious. He quotes Sir Arthur Eddington:

> [I]n the world of physics we watch a shadow graph performance of familiar life. The shadow of my elbow rests on the shadow table as the shadow-ink flows over the shadow paper; . . . the frank realization that physical science is concerned with a whole of a shadow is one of the most significant in recent advances.[50]

This, then, is the key: a mechanistic science is too limited; too many phenomena do not "fit" its idioms of explanation. Many scientists refuse to examine the shifting and flimsy base upon which they stand. For centuries man has used carefully constructed filters to deflect certain data that did not fit prevailing paradigms. Information has been ignored because it threatened the premises of the existing scientific enterprise, or because it was generated by suspect investigators. But given the steady accumulation of evidence of paranormal phenomena, the filters will have to be changed and the paradigms altered—and this is as true of medicine as it is of physics.[51]

Interconnectedness. For centuries we have assumed that we were a species apart, creatures of a different order and type, unrelated to other life forms. Modern medicine has built upon this premise by isolating patients for treatment, but worse, by isolating patients from their environments. We live in a complex network of interactions—we are not a shielded, invulnerable species. There are many examples.

It is possible to construct a pyramid with the proportion base to sides of 15.7 to 14.94, with a height of 10 of the same units. If oriented so that base lines face magnetic north-south and east-west, a used razor blade placed within and along the axis east-west can be resharpened indefinitely.

Nelya Mikhailova[52] and Uri Geller have little in common except one thing: telepathic and psychokinetic capabilities. Nelya is an elderly Russian housewife; Geller, a young Israeli. Mikhailova can move small objects short distances at will without touching them, although with great exertion. Geller can do that and more.

Even the most recalcitrant physician is coming to the realization that acupuncture works. What is known repudiates the "specific" theory of pain which is incorporated into Western medical practice. But beyond that our knowledge is slender. All that is clear is that acupuncturists trigger pain-blocking mechanisms in the body through the isolation of points for the insertion and manipulation of needles. How these points were discovered is veiled in history. However, on the assumption that trial and error would have been inefficient (and perhaps painful), it is possible that the body signals its vulnerabilities, that it can cause alterations in its energy field.

The work of Harold Burr of the Yale School of Medicine and Cleve Backster has demonstrated an "energy field" or aura that surrounds the body. In *The Fields of Life: Our Links With the Universe,*[53] Burr reports fluctuations in the body's energy field at ovulation, and abnormalities in the fields of women with cancer of the cervix. Backster's work has been mainly with plants. He has demonstrated their receptivity to stimuli measured first with a polygraph and more recently with an electroencephalogram.[54] He has also recorded plant responses to verbal threats, to the boiling of briny shrimp, and in more recent experiments, unfertilized egg "responses" to the impending and actual boiling of a fellow egg.[55]

Astrology has never been fashionable among intellectuals. In its routine application its claims are often preposterous. But there is some evidence that its premises may be sound, however much it is inflated in practice. A handful of recent studies reveal statistically significant correlations between "cosmic" events and human behavior. For example, in a study of more than 500,000 births in New York hospitals between 1948 and 1957, there was a clear and unmistakable trend for more births to occur during a waxing rather than waning moon. The sun may have even more impact. Data on traffic accidents in both Russia and Germany demonstrate that more accidents, as many as four times more, occur on the day following solar flare eruptions as on other days. Psychiatric admissions show a similar trend.[56]

The most provocative evidence has been compiled by Michael Gauquelin of the psychophysiological laboratory at Strasbourg. In *The Cosmic Clocks,*[57] Gauquelin summarizes more than 20 years of research on sidereal phenomena. His initial work focused on the relationship between the rise of the planets Mars and Saturn at the time of the birth of children who subsequently became successful physicians. The results were statistically significant; the chance odds are roughly 10 million to one. Gauquelin's subsequent work has added to the record. Correlations have been found with the ascendancy of Mars for soldiers, athletes, and politicians. Writers, painters, and musicians are negatively correlated with the influence of Mars and Saturn but positively with no other configuration.

Gauquelin's work may be a classic example of misplaced concreteness. Moreover, research of this sort should be challenged and more should be done. The point is that prevailing explanations do not and cannot contain the results. As Gunther Stent, a biologist at Stanford, pointed out in *Scientific American*,[58] telepathy, precognition, and psychokinesis breach elementary physical laws, and hence do not "fit" the traditional means of explaining things.

In *Supernature*,[59] Lyall Watson, a biologist and zoologist, discusses most the studies of paranormal phenomena mentioned in this chapter. *Supernature* is a survey of the literature and research focused on the interconnectedness of humanity and the rest of nature. As Watson says:

> Too often we see only what we expect to see: our view of the world is restricted by the blinkers of our limited experience, but it need not be this way. Supernature is nature with all its flavors intact waiting to be tasted. I offer it as a logical extension of the present state of science as a solution to some of the problems with which traditional science cannot cope and as an analgesic to modern man.
>
> I hope that it will prove to be more than that. Few aspects of human behavior are so persistent as our need to believe in things unseen—and as a biologist, I find it hard to accept that this is purely fortuitous. The belief, or the strange things to which this belief is so stubbornly attached, must have real survival value, and I think that we are rapidly approaching a situation in which this value will become apparent. As man uses up the resources of the world, he is going to have to rely more and more on his own. Many of these are at the moment concealed in the occult—a word that simply means "secret knowledge" and is a very good description of something that we have known all along but have been hiding from ourselves.[60]*

The strength of *Supernature* lies as much in its critical stance as in its comprehensiveness. As a primer to the student of the occult, in the sense of secret or unknown science,

---

the book is unprecedented. But Watson is also a scientist —his agnosticism transforms the book into something more than occult gossip. Watson continuously exposes the reader to his doubts and reflections, while stopping short of slamming doors. An example is his discussion of ghosts and communications with the dead:

> Communications with the dead are . . . suspect. I cannot help wondering why, out of the billions who once walked the earth, it should always be Napoleon, Shakespeare, Tolstoy, Chopin, Cleopatra, Robert Browning, and Alexander the Great who just happen to be on hand when a spirit medium summons up someone from the past. Rhine, the pioneer of parapsychological research in the United States, sums up the problem by saying, "The outcome of the scientific investigation of mediumship is best described as a draw." In seventy-five years of research no incontestable proof of survival has been found, but neither has it been possible to prove that some sort of survival after death could not occur.[61]*

His summary of psychokinesis is similar:

> The role of sympathetic magic and of superstition in psychokinetic phenomena is undoubtedly a large one, but I believe that, even without those props, we now have enough evidence to warrant the serious consideration of PK as a biological reality. There is a long way to go before we understand how it works, but we can already begin to think about its evolutionary implications. In man the ability seems to be manifest mainly in children, or essentially childlike personalities, and then most often as a casual, almost accidental effect. It is apparently important to believe that the mind can influence matter, or at least not to disbelieve it can. This suggests that its origins lie in some more primitive condition, which is preserved in the unconscious and later smothered by acquired cultural and intellectual pressures. But learning to produce PK effects on demand, by a conscious physical process, is probably a new development altogether.[62]*

* *From Supernature* by Lyall Watson. Copyright © 1973 by Lyall Watson. Used by permission of Doubleday & Company, Inc.

The implications of this research are fascinating. One area to which the research points is brain wave studies. The rates and rhythms of brain waves are well established. But to discover something more than rate fluctuations due to normal stimuli such as drugs and sleep, more penetrating experiments were designed. Gray Walter, a British neurophysiologist, has explored the relationship between epilepsy and brain wave frequencies. He found that spontaneous seizures could be induced in known epileptics by flashing light into the subject's eyes at alpha-rhythm range—roughly 8 to 12 cycles per second. He then found that about 1 of 20 persons who had never experienced a seizure responded, some spasmodically, some with nausea, to light flickers trained on their eye surfaces.

This research was extended by others into analyses of the impact of other frequencies and in particular "infrasounds"—frequencies at less than 10 to 20 cycles per second—below the threshold of human hearing. As with many other recent discoveries, the initial revelation arose by chance. Professor Gavraud from Marseilles always felt ill at work, not an unusual experience. But Gavraud, a curious and diligent worker, decided to find out why he was always sick. After some false starts he located the trouble—his office was vibrating at a low frequency as a result of the thrum of an air conditioner unit on top of the building directly across the street. The rhythm—7 cycles per second—made him ill.

The cause of Gavraud's nausea has been confirmed by other studies. Low frequency sound waves do affect the body, and in some cases illness can result.[63] But Gavraud did not stop there. Perplexed by the phenomenon, he built a 6-foot whistle, powered with compressed air and modeled after the whistle carried by French gendarmes. It is not known whether Gavraud had taken out the French equivalent of workmen's compensation coverage, but one can only hope so because the technician Gavraud enlisted to aid him in the first trial with the superwhistle expired on the spot when it was blown. In later, more carefully controlled work, Gavraud only succeeded in shattering windows.[64]

We take light for granted, but there is more than one kind of light. Most of us, since we live and work in artificial environments, are constantly exposed to artificial light. But the principal theme in John Ott's *Health and Light*[65] is that natural light is healthier. Ott gets to this conclusion through some studies; unfortunately, few are rigorously empirical. In one of the more thorough studies, Ott investigated the influence of wave lengths of light on spontaneous tumor development in C_3H mice. Figure 13 is reproduced from *Health and Light*.

Ott has also looked at human responses to light. His work thus far is provocative. For example, he reports on a potential relationship between the use of full-spectrum lighting —rarely used in commerce today—and the contraction of flu:

> During the winter of 1968–1969 a serious outbreak of Hong Kong flu swept the country. Florida was no exception. The Health Department reported 5 percent of Sarasota County—or 6,000 people—sick with the flu at one time. Employee illness caused the temporary closing of one supermarket, a social club, and the shutdown of two areas of the Sarasota Memorial Hospital because sixty-one nurses were out with the flu.
>
> Obrig Laboratories, located just north of Sarasota, is one of the largest manufacturers of contact lenses and has approximately one hundred employees. During the entire flu epidemic not one employee was absent because of any flu type ailment, according to Philip Salvatori, Chairman of the Board.
>
> Obrig Laboratories was the first to design a new building using full-spectrum lighting and ultraviolet-transmitting plastic panes throughout the entire office and factory areas. The added ultraviolet seemed to tie in closely with the results noted at the "Well of the Sea" restaurant in Chicago. Mr. Salvatori also mentioned that the Obrig employees had not been given any mass inoculation against the Hong Kong flu, although some individuals may have received shots from their private physicians. Mr. Salvatori also commented that everyone seemed

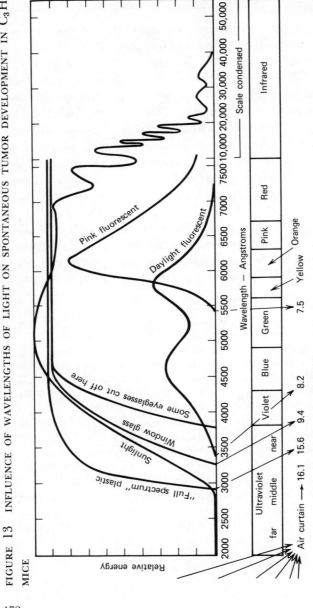

FIGURE 13 INFLUENCE OF WAVELENGTHS OF LIGHT ON SPONTANEOUS TUMOR DEVELOPMENT IN C₃H MICE

Note. Mercury vapor lines in fluorescent lights have been omitted. John Ott, *Health and Light* (Old Greenwich, Ct.: Devin Adair, Publishers); by permission of Devin Adair.

172

happier and in better spirits under the new lighting, and that work production had increased by at least 25 percent.[66]

Ott's work may have established a link between the nature and quality of light exposure and health status. Unfortunately, he has yet to conduct sufficiently rigorous work. But, at a minimum, his work should elicit more work.

If the preservation of perishables is possible in pyramids and cyclical frequencies of light and sound affect man, the implications for health are enormous. Today, the physician's armamentarium is limited to sharp instruments, pills, and cryptic advice. Professor Gavraud could have swallowed hundreds of pills and had a frontal lobotomy and still felt ill. How many infrasounds pulse through the average hospital stuffed with sophisticated apparatus? What do physicians do about light?

These questions are rhetorical, and perhaps unfair. Hospitals and physicians do not concern themselves with sound and light because they perceive different problems and undertake different missions. But that is the point: They provide medical care, and only incidentally does that result in health.

Much of the research on interconnectedness is inexplicable; we have done little work so far, and we consequently know very little. But this much is clear: Explanations of human life in parochial and mechanistic terms will have to be modified, if not abandoned. Man is inextricably a part of his world and of a cosmic order. The signs are becoming abundant. Aside from the mysticism that always dances at the edge of accepted knowledge, we have generally constructed explanations of how things work out of our material and social environment. Western intellectual history is a canvas with man at the center. The demonology of Hieronymus Bosch was only a slice of the hell below us. The spirituality of Michelangelo is soaring, but at the same time earthbound, as if the gods were etched into an impermeable umbrella just

a few miles above us. Our demonic and spiritual imagery
—our religious expressions—have been decidedly an-
thropocentric. We assumed that our world is our sandbox. If
there are "gods" we assume they have long since written us
off, and we they. Our sense of oneness with the rest of our
world and beyond has been truncated; and correspondingly,
our sense of reality has been tragically limited.

Overproduction of Services.   It is common in economic theory
to refer to "externalities" in the production of material
goods. (An "externality" is thought of as a by-product of the
production process and can be viewed as either a "good" or
"bad" result, or as external economy or external dis-
economy.) In production processes, externalities include
water and air pollution, noise, and in a more concrete sense,
black-lung disease among coal miners. But in the conventional view, while there can be too many products and unfortunately byproducts in the form of externalities as well, it
is not generally thought that services generate externalities.

One of the reasons the idea is novel derives from the
"politics" of services. Services—health care, legal advice,
education, welfare, and social aides—are designed to support those whose lack of material or human resources renders them vulnerable to the depredations of a competitive
culture. In this sense services are society's answer to the
failure to ensure economic equality—equality of opportunity
is the catchword. Equality is possible only if services can be
delivered to ensure that the "disadvantaged" have a fighting
chance. Given this conceptualization of services, it follows
that as long as there are those who remain in need, services
cannot be overproduced.

There are at least three reasons why this view is in error.
First, it presupposes that the recipient benefits from services.
This is a highly controversial issue and one that deserves far
more sophisticated treatment than I can give it here. There

are instances of "benefits": the child who learns to read, the mother who "grows" when her children are placed in a day care program, and the family that utilizes "well-baby" care. But in the aggregate and in the long run there is doubt that services accomplish the purposes for which they were designed. In education, for example, a string of major studies, including the Coleman report and *Inequality* by Christopher Jencks and others,[67] demonstrate that schooling fails to achieve one of its major purposes—the economic success of its graduates. The Coleman and Jencks studies are surrounded by controversy, but their conclusions have yet to be refuted.

The failure of the services strategy to remedy poverty has been argued by many. There are few who do not think that the current welfare services system is a shambles. The failure of welfare reform is not testimony to the strength of the current welfare system, but rather to the political troglodytes who have opposed change.

The point is that while some may benefit, services are not always unmitigated blessings.

The second reason is related to the first. The original purpose of services was to create a climate where the vulnerable could become self-sufficient. But the opposite has occurred—services have created and now maintain millions in dependency. The "vicious cycle of poverty" has not been checked, much less broken. More than two million people are on welfare in New York City alone. While education has paved the way to material rewards for many, many others lack the most basic survival skills. These include those who simply did not and could not learn, as well as those whose need for skills did not match what the schools were selling. Finally, we are *all* dependent on health services and therapy. We do not pursue health and well-being—we try to avoid sickness. And that is precisely what medicine has taught us to do.

Supply and demand lies at the root of the third point. In

all service sectors, large, complex, expensive, and unwieldy bureaucracies have prospered and grown at the expense of those in need. For this reason dependency and need cannot disappear—they are necessary functional attributes of a service economy. If all of the criminal statutes on the books in the United States were repealed tomorrow, save one, almost any one, the next day roughly the same number of people would be snared for the one crime as may otherwise have been apprehended for the hundreds of crimes now on the books. Services create their own demand, and if that demand is greater than it should be, then those services are overproduced.

Much of this analysis is indebted to Ivan Illich, who first in *Deschooling Society*,[68] but more trenchantly in *Tools for Conviviality*,[69] develops the thesis of overproduction. Illich uses health and medicine to illustrate the latter work. In simple form his argument is that the institutions of medicine pursue their own objectives—security, growth, stability, and income—and as such *must* create widespread dependency on the part of a consuming public. This necessarily results in stripping the tools for health from the people and restricting their use to those who have been certified. Illich characterizes medicine's aggrandizement by alluding to two watersheds: the first in 1913 when it first began to borrow from the scientific method, and the second in 1955 when it first became clear that medicine created new forms of disease —iatrogenic disorders—in its frenzied efforts to cure. But Illich does not single out medicine:

> Other industrial institutions have passed through the same two watersheds. This is certainly true for the major social agencies that have been reorganized according to scientific criteria during the last 150 years. Education, the mails, social work, transportation, and even civil engineering have followed this evolution. At first, new knowledge is applied to the solution of a clearly stated problem and scientific measuring sticks are applied to account for the new efficiency. But at a second point, the progress demonstrated in a previous achievement is used as a

rationale for the exploitation of society as a whole in the service of a value which is determined and constantly revised by an element of society, by one of its self-certifying professional elites.[70]

Death. Along with taxes, death is supposed to be inevitable, and it is; but in contemporary society medicine's chief task has been the prolongation of life. Grappling with death is not an easy matter—medicine expends a staggering amount of resources in doing so. Robert M. Hutchins, Chairman of the Center for the Study of Democratic Institutions, referring to his own treatment, pointed out that the resources lavished on him "could have wiped out cholera in South Asia."

Cultural views of death have changed radically over the centuries. To greatly oversimplify, our contemporary conception of death has become more fearful and more dread as the cushions of religion, family, and ritual have failed. In the past, death was simply a feature of life—it was frequent, inevitable, and could not be postponed. Socioreligious beliefs fostered the notion that death was certain and arrived at a fixed time for everyone. But soon some slippage occurred. Because of improved living conditions, a few people survived the subsistence economy and entered old age without having succumbed to the rigors of work. Having made it that far, and occasionally possessing the resources to buy the help to survive longer, they sought life-prolonging aid. And thus a new social role was created—the physician whose task it was to prolong life and frustrate death.[71] In this way the physician's role was distinguishable from that of the shaman. In most early cultures the shaman's task was not to defeat death, but to ease the passage from life to death. The rituals distracted the patient's attention from the disease affecting him. If remissions occurred, it was more than likely due to the patient's will to live abetted by the mind-set achieved with the help of the shaman.[72]

Life is less dangerous today. With the improvement in living conditions death is not as swift and certain as it once was. Correspondingly, the physician's role has enlarged. There is

no longer such a thing as a "natural" death. Death must be
clinically categorized—it must be "caused" by some clinical
condition for which treatment can or could have been prescribed. Medicine's purveyance of health as a good is then
matched by its "control" over death—its "sale" of life. So the
paradox deepens: Medicine deals in disease by selling units of
health, and deals with death by selling life. But in neither case
is the patient given responsibility for the result.

Elisabeth Kübler-Ross, M.D., in *On Death and Dying*,[73] depicts the struggle between the dying patient and death. She
indicts the medical profession for its treatment of the dying.
The physician is as uncomfortable around death as anyone
and most often deals with it callously, but it is the physician
who has arrogated the position of death-defier. But death is
a natural condition, as well as a date that can be put off. To
the extent medicine does something other than delay the
inevitable with drugs and machines, it has a proper role. But
it sells life by promising miracles; in fact, it does little more
than delay death. Most of the dying are in degenerating
states due to the ravages of disease caused by poor health
habits, age, and occasionally trauma. Medicine cannot cure
these conditions; but in its marketing of life, it simultane-
ously invades the province of "natural" death. The thing
most dying people want is to be in a familiar place with
loving people. But because of medicine's control over death,
the patient is wired, doped, and incarcerated in a sterile
hospital room surrounded by indifference.

The "right to die" is slowly gaining force. The recognition
will dawn that medicine cannot cure death and that spontaneous remissions of terminal illness are the product of the
patient's will to live.

Two tasks remain. First, since so much time has been
spent saying what health is not, something should be said
about what health is. And then, as a second task, building
upon these concepts, a new medicine can be constructed.

6

What Then Is Health?

> My father . . . went to Paris and became solicitor to the British
> Embassy. . . . After my mother's death, her maid became my
> nurse. . . . I think my father had a romantic mind. He took it into
> his head to build a house to live in during the summer. He bought
> a piece of land on top of a hill at Suresnes. . . . It was to be like a
> villa on the Bosphorus and on the top floor it was surrounded by
> loggias. . . . It was a white house and the shutters were painted
> red. The garden was laid out. The rooms were furnished, and
> then my father died.
>
> Somerset Maugham, *The Summing Up*

Thus far I have tried to demonstrate that medicine has little to
do with health. But then what does? Unfortunately, we do not
know much. Our preoccupation with the provision of services
has precluded analysis of the factors conducive to health. We
have spent so much time defining and classifying the sick and
sicknesses that we have learned very little about health and the
healthy. Nevertheless, we do know a few things, and we can
build upon them while we try to find out more.

Health, like disease, is the result of many factors. This is a
deceptively simple statement. Perhaps the greatest debt we
owe to René Dubos lies in his recognition that the cause of
disease is multiple. For decades (and in some backwaters
today) it was assumed that disease was caused by a "single
bullet," a single cause. This is the premise of the germ theory of
disease, patiently constructed by such pioneers as Pasteur,
Koch, and Lister.[1]

Dubos acknowledges that there is a physiological basis to disease, but he convincingly accounts for the greater impact of environmental and social factors. At times he comes close to attributing disease solely to extraphysiological factors, but stopping short, ultimately he provides the foundation for our emerging understanding of disease. In simple terms, every person carries the potential for every disease at all times. But through circumstances that vary with every individual, some people get sick while others, similarly situated, do not. This is not the same thing as saying that disease has no physical base. Rather, the physical base for disease, which probably varies with the nature of the disease, must be triggered by events external to the individual.

A logical extension of this theory is that some people "select" diseases (or injuries) because they find illness preferable to stress.[2] This is exemplified by the work of some sociologists, most notably Talcott Parsons, on sick roles. To Parsons and others, some individuals choose or are forced to choose to play a sick role in given social settings.[3]

But Dubos's theory only accounts for disease. What are the implications for a different understanding of health? To Dubos they are clear: Because a human being is the subject of many changing and inevitable demands and stresses, medicine can never produce health through its focus on specific disease conditions. There is no ultimate cure for disease. A disease-free world is impossible:

> The concept of perfect and positive health is a utopian creation of the mind. It cannot become reality because man will never be so perfectly adapted to his environment that his life will not involve struggles, failures, and sufferings. . . . The less pleasant reality is that in an ever-changing world each period and each type of civilization will continue to have its burden of disease created by the unavoidable failures of adaptation to the new environment.[4]

The human is a complex of physiological and social roles and is continuously subject to social and environmental stresses. Consequently, to Dubos a healthy society is one in which the natural adaptability of the species is enhanced, not one in which disease does not exist. Health then is maximum adaptability to the inevitability of disease.

The limitation of Dubos's analysis lies in its stress on disease. This is true of most definitions of health. Health is more than the absence of disease—in fact, it often cohabits with disease. A person with diabetes or with a heart murmur is not sick but merely a different person—one with certain constraints. But such a person can be as healthy within those limits as anyone else. Health is a positive state. For decades attempts have been made to generate a positive definition of health. The World Health Organization definition is generally considered to be the most comprehensive: "A state of complete physical and mental well-being and not merely the absence of disease or infirmity." But the definition does not go far enough. Most definitions of health which seek to go beyond the absence of disease focus on functional capacity—health is said to be that state in which the individual can function. Functional capacity is important and basic to health, but it too is insufficient.

There are two deficiencies underlying most definitions of health, including WHO's. First, health is too frequently measured against some objective and extrinsic standard such as the absence of pathology, the capacity to function in a given social role, or the freedom from disability. Second, health is erroneously conceived of as a state or property of an organism rather than as a dynamic condition, a constantly evolving source of energy.

Because of these deficiencies, current conceptualizations of health have inculcated a deep dependence on the part of the public: a dependence on the social setting for definitions of health synonymous with functioning in that setting, and an even more profound dependence on services to produce states of health. This dependency, which feeds the growth of the medical care system, also frustrates the conceptualization of new approaches to health. Health is a dynamic state, one the individual can actively pursue. But even this is not all there is to it. Certain conditions lie beyond the reach of the individual. So health then is a mix of social and environmental contexts conducive to health and individual behavior and choice consistent with those contexts. How does all of this fit together?

FOUR CONDITIONS OF HEALTH

Any new approach to or reconceptualization of health must be based on four attributes or conditions: a harmonious socioenvironment, readily obtainable resources to aid in becoming and staying healthy, someone to care, and individual responsibility.

The Social and Environmental Context. There is abundant evidence that social and environmental factors singly and in combination frustrate and even prevent individuals from maintaining their health. People are not born ill; even those with congenital defects can be healthy. But as interactions with a degraded physical environment and a perverted social order multiply, disease is often the result. Trees and shrubs that flourish in other settings become ragged and thin and often die when they border a heavily traveled road. The natural condition of life is to thrive—to fulfill a phenotypical ideal. But the maturation of an organism can be stunted and warped by a debilitating environment. The cigarette smoker, the coal miner, the alcoholic, and angry and hostile businessmen all have one thing in common: They are steadily broken by their environment. Each loses measurable amounts of life and vitality each day. But it is not the physical environment alone that can be unhealthy; the social order contains pathology as well. The child who is repeatedly told that genitalia are "dirty" may fulfill the parental prophecy by contracting a venereal disease.

Man and the rest of nature are inextricably interconnected. For centuries human beings have tried to subjugate the environment to their will. But, as Gregory Bateson remarks, "the creature that wins against its environment destroys itself."[5] Our approach to health mirrors this distortion. We have failed to think about disease and health in symbiotic terms. We view disease as a thing apart—not another constituent of nature but an implacable enemy. Our approach has been warfare. We seek to suppress disease, to crush it with drugs, to burn it with lasers, and to cut it out with surgical tools.

But, as Dubos has argued, most of us carry most diseases most of the time, in the sense that we carry the ingredients of disease with us. Some diseases are communicated, but many diseases or illnesses, possibly including the communicable ills, occur only when our susceptibility increases. Disease reflects imbalances within us, as well as between us and the external world. To deal only with the symptoms of the imbalance, the disharmony, is like retreading a tire, or drinking alcohol to "cure" a hangover. The treatment of symptoms alone is unadulterated expediency. Unless the context is treated—unless the environment is made safe for us to live in and our social order transformed to foster health—we shall remain sick.

Resources. In *The Well Body Book,*[6] a treatise on self-care, the authors entitle one chapter "Your Doctor as a Resource." Until their apotheosis this was what doctors were; they did not have much knowledge and their tools were limited, but they came when they were asked and they helped as much by their presence as by their skill. Today, we, the patients, have become the resource—without us the doctors cannot function. So we do what we are told, and we insistently return for more of the same. But even assuming a happy social order and an optimal environment, and even assuming that individuals understood their bodies, help would still be needed. Not all people can set a bone as ably as someone trained to do it. Someone else might know more about medications; a third might possess diagnostic skills. Moreover, for certain afflictions a place of peace and quiet, like a hospital, might be instrumental in restoring health. So even with the best of air and water, reductions of stress, and wider and deeper knowledge of the initiatives necessary to maintain health, resources must be available. Not everyone can or should care for themselves and many might be unable to care for others. Health care resources will be needed but they should be just that—resources available to those who need them.

"Caring."   There is a danger in forcing medicine to meet too rigorous a test. If medicine is measured only by its clinical effectiveness, that is, whether the processes used by physicians have anything to do with the outcome to the patient, much of what is done now may be discarded. Although much should be discarded while the house is being cleaned and the rummage sale held, care must be taken not to throw out too much. As I have pointed out, many office visits are just that—visits. In an age of alienation and isolation, many need someone to turn to for care and for help. Home care may compare favorably with hospital care, even for some acute conditions, precisely because caring is maximized in the home.

But to retain caring in the medicine of the future does not require us to mortgage ourselves today. A smaller, leaner medical care system can still care. In addition, health science students could be selected for their capacity to care and heal, rather than for their quantitative skills, dexterity, and efficiency. Caring should be a part of the medicine of tomorrow.

The Individual. The most important factor in health is the individual who desires to be healthy. The role of the individual in the current system is negligible. But despite almost palpable dependency there are some whose will to be healthy overcomes both their pathology and the attempts to heal them. There are some who understand their bodies. Theodore Roszak refers to this kind of knowledge as "that [which] must come through the body and be accepted on the body's own terms as a lesson not to be learned elsewhere or otherwise: an organic message, organically integrated."[7]

It is surprising how much health is an intuitional matter. I recently traveled to Mexico. Like many other North Americans, I became a victim of "Montezuma's revenge." For a stretch of about 48 hours, I was genuinely ill, but the experience also revealed that acute perception of the body's workings is possible. Almost as a diversion, I monitored the battle within me; I tried to sense and get in touch with what my body was doing to deal with the imbalance. I took some pills and drank some herbal tea proffered to me by a sympathetic native. And it worked temporarily. But I knew the imbalance would remain and would take weeks to redress, even though the most severe symptoms would disappear in a few days. Since that time I have paid more attention to the many signals I get from my body. The body signals as surely as an onrushing train. All of us have felt cravings for certain kinds of foods at certain times. Pregnant women often change their diets because their bodies signal for different nutrients. But we have to listen. In a small and simple way it is one of the methods to be healthy.

There are other signals, often less detectable. Transcontinental and intercontinental travelers are out of phase with their normal environments on arrival. This often accounts for the extraordinary fatigue and poor performance that affect many travelers, most of whom try to resist. The body is a creature of patterns and cycles. Certain fixed rhythms and cycles are rooted in our history and biology. Gay Gaer Luce in *Body Time*[8] reviews the research that has been done on the sensitivity of the body to time—how mood, performance, activity, and tactility all fluctuate in an elaborate dance with time:

> Time is the most intimate and pervasive aspect of our lives, yet the language of our self-expectations is static. We traverse the life cycle from birth to maturity, aging, and death. We observe the round of seasons, the ceaseless alternation of day and night. We are touched by inner cycles of sleepiness and hunger, yet our self-image is as fixed as a photograph. We expect consistent feeling and behavior in family and friends. We aspire to undeviating performance at work, and measure our state of health against some static norm. Our habitual language imposes the expectations of a steady state. All of this hinders us from feeling our rhythmic nature.[9]

There is a rich mine of literature on this subject. The human organism exists in a pulsating web of interactions with other animate life, with terrestrial and solar waves and radiations, and with man-made machines and equipment. Most interactions take place at subconscious levels. The human animal throbs at its own rates, and projects, as well as receives, impulses. The health of an individual depends on the calibration of external impulses and signals with internal rhythms and messages.

In all developed countries male death rates are substantially higher than those of females of comparable ages. At all ages, the unmarried have considerably higher death rates than the married. And in Nevada, infant mortality is 40 percent higher than in Utah and contiguous states.[10] There are many partial explanations: Mormons neither consume the alcohol nor inhale the cigarette smoke that hovers over the populated parts of Nevada, heart disease selectively affects males in developed countries, and so on. But why do the unmarried die earlier? One important factor is that the married want to live more.[11] The individual will to be well is critical. Diet, nutrition, exercise, rest, and calm all make a difference, as do doctors, but the healthy individual must make choices and must be informed in order to do so.

There are two kinds of knowledge. There is a need for information—what to do about one signal or another, when to ask for help, what kind of food to eat to ensure a sufficient amount of energy, and so on. But of equal importance is experiential knowledge—body consciousness—the capacity to read the topography of feelings and sensations. The first can be taught to some extent; the second can only be experienced. The second takes nothing less than the assumption by the individual of the responsibility for health, and concomitantly an escape from a dependency on others. A healer can only help to restore health and maintain it. The individual is chiefly responsible.

In *Fear and Trembling*,[12] Sören Kierkegaard describes the "man of faith." The man of faith, far from being a man of heroic proportions, is indistinguishable from anyone else. He walks home from work puffing on his pipe, pauses to watch a construction project, arrives at home, rests, and eats his lamb chops for dinner and retires soon thereafter. Similarly, the healthy person is not distinctive or readily distinguishable. The pursuit of health is not limited to heroes. Although we know little about health, what we do know is easy to execute and is largely dependent on the individual.

BIOMEDICAL RESOURCES FOR HEALTH

In this book I have discussed factors and behaviors that evidence indicates are related to health. They include exercise, nutrition, and food contaminants, clear air and water, noise levels, dirt, waste material, stress and congestion, light and sound, housing, rest, choices and opportunities, recreation, motivation, attitude and assumption of responsibility, healing and the symbols of healing, and medical care resources. In each case there is some evidence of a relationship to health; and in some cases more than others. But with rare exceptions we have no information about their *relative* importance. Nevertheless, we have lavished almost all of the health dollar on medical care and starved the rest. A better balance must be struck.

It costs about $2800 to install an artificial plastic and steel ball-and-socket hip joint in an arthritic patient.[13] Since arthritis is a common ailment of old age, it follows that many will desire the implantation of artificial joints and sockets. But who will get new hips or new knuckles; only the rich? Will Medicare pay for new hips for thousands at the cost of millions? I do not know the answers, but the questions are forced by the availability of technology—services cannot be withheld from those who can afford them. But the availability of technology also results in consumption of funds otherwise available to attack other problems in other ways. The choices are hard to make, but today no choices are offered. As long as the technology is available, it will be implemented—who can deny relief to the sick? As a result we continue in our ignorance of the potential benefits of programs that are nonmedical in nature and of the relative importance of various programs, including medical care.

The solution is not simple. People cannot be bludgeoned into positive health habits. But if it is true that biomedical technology drives the system, then a shift in biomedical research priorities may be a key. If we want to know more about light, nutrition, and recreation and less about artificial knuckle joints we should pay for the former and not the latter. Nutrition is a good example. We know next to nothing about it—we know that a papaya is probably better for us than a Hostess Twinky, but that is about it. Physicians do not know much about it either and consequently do not think it important. And because they think it unimportant, few research monies are available. To quote Roger J. Williams, the discoverer of a key B vitamin, "There is not a shadow of a doubt . . . that medical science has neglected nutrition to the point of disaster."[14]

So it is a question of emphasis—emphasis on medical care to the exclusion of other factors. The emphasis has been on the treatment of disease, not on the promotion of health.

THE PROMOTION OF HEALTH

It is misleading to define "health" as a state, or as a product of anterior activities and services. Health is a dynamic process. To think of health in this way is to reflect the knowledge implicit in an ecological world view. The passing view—derived ·largely from a mechanistic world view —assumes that human beings and nature are competitors and hence that human survival is dependent on control and manipulation of nature. This is also the premise of modern medicine. Disease and sickness are losses to nature; they occur when the body has been invaded by agents of disease. And correspondingly, the fight against disease incorporates military metaphors: The surgeon "attacks" the body and "removes" the disease; drugs are administered to blunt the disease agent and "vanquish" it. But given the complexity of man's relationship to nature—the ecology of life—it is increasingly clear that health does not result from winning a war. The radical view of the world that ecology compels also compels a radical view of health since health is neither a cause nor an effect, but a dynamic condition, one that both acts and is acted upon.[15]

In a powerful paper, "Health and Healthing: Beyond Disease and Dysfunctional Environments,"[16] Bob Hoke, a medical corpsman at the Naval Medical Research Institute of the National Naval Medical Center, has begun the job of rethinking health. In striving for new thinking about health,

Hoke relies on John Dewey, particularly on his book, *Knowing and the Known*,[17] where Dewey stresses a "transactional" view. This view emphasizes interdependence and complementarity, even synchronicity, as opposed to causal relations. In terms of health, to quote Hoke, "the transactional imagination suggests a shift from viewing individuals as the only units for diagnosis, treatment and prevention of disease to observing the specific *situations* of a man-environment transaction" (emphasis in original). Following this conceptualization, disease is a symptom or signal of a dysfunctional "man-environment transaction," and the "situation" for treating the disease *and* promoting health. It is for this reason that Hoke rejects the use of the word "health" as a noun, and prefers a verb, "healthing." Fredrick Sargent puts it this way:

> It is unreasonable to think of health as a characteristic of the man *per se*. Because man and environment constitute a system, health is a process of man-environment interaction within a particular ecological context.[18]

To think of health this way does not entail dividing the sick and the well into separate camps. Health and disease are not separate states or qualities. We do not move from one state to another as if changing clothes. Rather, health and disease are part of a process or continuum, "mutually interdependent aspects of a situation." As I have said, the sick can be healthy, or as Hoke puts it, "There is a healthy way to live a disease."[19]

But to view health this way does compel us to devote at least equal attention to the characteristics of health and the healthy; and probably more attention, since the classifications of disease have been the exclusive preoccupation of medicine. And it leads as well to viewing "healthing" in behavioral terms. If this is so, treating sickness and promoting health both require a thorough examination of the environmental and social constraints to healthy behavior. This is more than "population" medicine; it is more than garbage pickup and potable water. The promotion of health includes these measures, but also requires reconstruction of the behavioral environment in which a person lives in order to facilitate healthing. This may include the treatment of illness, but it also embraces changes in personal, social, and environmental contexts. People must choose to be healthy by acting healthy. And we must also rearrange our social and environmental orders to foster health.

Many of these ideas seem commonsensical, but it is surprising how little recognition they are given. Recently, however, the Canadian government has addressed the issues head-on. In *A New Perspective on the Health of Canadians,* a publication of the Government of Canada, the limits of medical care to produce health are expressly acknowledged, and the role of social, environmental, and personal factors is recognized. The report does not equivocate.

> The health care system, however, is only one of many ways of maintaining and improving health. Of equal or greater importance in increasing the number of illness-free days in the lives of Canadians have been the raising of the general standard of living, important sanitary measures for protecting public health, and advances in medical science.

> At the same time as improvements have been made in health care, in the general standard of living, in public health protection and in medical science, ominous counter-forces have been at work to undo progress in raising the health status of Canadians. These counter-forces constitute the dark side of economic progress. They include environmental pollution, city living, habits of indolence, the abuse of alcohol, tobacco and drugs, and eating patterns which put the pleasing of the senses above the needs of the human body.

> For these environmental and behavioural threats to health, the organized health care system can do little more than serve as a catchment net for the victims. Physicians, surgeons, nurses and hospitals together spend much of their time in treating ills caused by adverse environmental factors and behavioural risks.

It is evident now that further improvements in the environment, reductions in self-imposed risks, and a greater knowledge of human biology are necessary if more Canadians are to live a full, happy, long and illness-free life.[20]

This is new language, but the concepts are not new. Rudolf Virchow, the "father of pathology" and a seminal figure in medicine, said in 1849:

In reality, if medicine is the science of the healthy as well as of the ill human being (which is what it ought to be), what other science is better suited to prepare laws as the basis of the social structure, in order to make effective those which are inherent in man himself? . . . Medicine is a social science in its very bone and marrow . . .[21]

Virchow also said, more trenchantly, "Medicine is nothing but a social science. Politics is nothing but medicine on a large scale."

7

The Transformations of Medicine

> Politics and economics are concerned with power and wealth, neither of which should be the primary, still less the exclusive, concern of full-grown men.
>
> Arthur C. Clarke, *Profiles of the Future*

Medicine has a history of scientific and social relations with society; it has always been practiced as an integral part of society.[1] But today medicine is insular. Today its politics are self-protective, its social posture defensive and conservative, and its modes of practice microscopic. Today medicine applies some theory, some empirics, and some hardware to increasingly smaller parts of the human machine. Today, even more than in the past, it focuses on the anatomy of the animal whose sickness has been inflicted by the environment in which he or she lives. But despite this, through professional dominance it has preserved and even expanded its jurisdiction over all things that it defines as "health." As Eliot Freidson says, "The medical profession has first claim to jurisdiction over the label of illness and *anything* to which it may be attached."[2]

Tomorrow, as society evolves, medicine will be even more myopic and more microscopic than it is now. Unless medicine is reexamined, the allocation of limited resources

will be made to perpetuate it, when a more rational allocation would contribute to the achievement of better health.

"THE TRAGEDY OF THE COMMONS"

The subtitle to the famous essay by Garrett Hardin, "The
Tragedy of the Commons" is, "The population problem has
no technical solution; it requires a fundamental extension in
morality."[3] To Hardin, the "tragedy of the commons" stems
from the incompatibility of individual choice and group survival. Each farmer with access to the commons gains by
increasing his use of it. If each individual increases his use of
it, the inevitable consequence is impoverishment for all as
the resources of the commons are depleted. Without a "new"
morality, the despoilation of the commons was inevitable.

The relationship of the consumer of medical care to the
medical care system is comparable to that of the farmer and
the commons, and the need for a new morality is equally
clear. There are finite limits to medical care, despite the
capacity of providers to stimulate demand and inflate supply
to staggering proportions.[4]

Health is no longer a condition. It is a commodity, a
unique and nonfungible good. Its transmogrification to a
commodity has been an inexorable process, but has accelerated in the last three or four decades. It has been a concomitant of the professionalization of providers, who are no
longer healers but sellers of goods chopped into units of
health. But there is a limit even to health "goods." The
demands of those with purchasing power and access cannot
be satisfied forever. And as the franchise has been extended
through Medicare and Medicaid, the seams of the system are
beginning to bulge. It now costs about $90 billion annually
to deliver the goods; in another few years it will cost more
than $100 billion, without a national health insurance pro-
gram. With national health insurance, costs will soar higher.[5]

Under these circumstances, how is the commons preserved? There are only two ways. The first—the route we are traveling—is to increase the number of suppliers, while fixing the "package" of "goods" which will be paid for by the government. (In this sense, the health commons is distinguishable to a degree from Hardin's commons—it is somewhat expandable, but not infinitely so.) In the simplest terms this solution, however appealing, will *not* lead to more health, no matter how many goods are ultimately delivered. This is because medical care—the goods to be delivered —does not produce much health, and, with the passage of time, will produce even less.

If the commons is thought of as the health of the population and not as a pool of goods to be parceled out by physicians, there is a second way to preserve it. This approach depends on a reconceptualization of health as something other than a commodity. When this is accomplished, a second step is possible: derivation of a program for the pursuit of health combining measures of individual responsibility, efficacious curative measures, and interventions into the environment. This is not an easy task; in fact because we know so little it is highly problematic. But if it is health we care about, rather than medical care, we must start. Before we start, however, we should briefly look at where we have been.

THE ERAS OF MEDICINE

Medicine began in mystery. But gradually measures were developed that worked, even if they were frequently bizarre. Blood was let in sacrifice, dances were danced, incantations were offered, and occasionally medicinals were used. And occasionally, the medicine of the past worked, often as not because the practitioner was perceptive and sensitive. But medicine still lacked a theoretical base—its successes were random.

Along the way, some galvanizing events occurred. The

first was the discovery that cleansing the environment
—developing sanitary sewage systems and improving the
potability of water—appeared to reduce mortality and morbidity. Thus, the sanitary services were slowly installed.

These services were significantly different from most
medicine; they were systemic and ecological in nature. They
were premised on interventions in the socioenvironment
rather than the human body. As such they were not measures that could be reduced to commodities rendered for
a price by healers to patients. Eventually, they were not
thought of as medical matters at all—they were decisions to
be made by the polity. Medical care, concomitantly, consisted
of healing those who were sick—why they were sick, or what
cured them if they were cured, was not necessarily relevant.
Thus, causes—the conditions and circumstances of life
—became divorced from effects. The effect—the sickness
and its symptoms—was what required treatment. Sickness
and its symptoms have been treated ever since, and causes
have been neglected.

A second pivotal event was the application of the scientific
method to medicine. Scientific methodology is a tool of great
utility, and scientific problem-solving found a congenial
home in medicine. Unlike other branches of science,
medicine possessed a captive supply of experimental subjects, and generally found revenue sources for biomedical
research easy marks.

It cannot be overemphasized that the application of
scientific methodology to healing produced substantial
benefits. It moved medicine out of the Middle Ages. But it
also demanded that medicine prove its effectiveness empiri-
cally. Medicine carried the burden of evidence for a few
decades. But the case is less convincing today, and will be
much harder to make in the future. The reason lies in
medicine's equation of reality with material reality. The emphasis in medicine on material reality—only what can be
perceived can be treated and only "symptoms" can be
perceived—has driven medicine to extremes.

In medicine, as well as in other disciplines, the pursuit of scientific purity results in reductionism of the subject matter. In part, the environmental crisis we face today stems from our inability to understand our world as an organism—as the spaceship Earth. In chemistry, in biology, and in medicine, increasingly investigators cannot communicate with one another because they have drawn rigid and narrow boundaries around their subjects. In medicine this has resulted in microscopism and specialization—with elegant empirical fireworks—on smaller and smaller parts of the human organism. When a physician let blood in the seventeenth century, he may not have benefited the patient much, but at least he perceived his patient as a single organism under the spell of some "humour." Today the physician removes a portion of the deteriorated stomach of an alcoholic patient and discharges the patient a few days later. The excised organ goes to the pathologist, the physician gets his or her fee, and the patient goes to the tavern.

A third transformation now faces medicine. Precisely at a time when it has achieved a feudal, even sovereign status—a state at great variance with its capacity to heal—shifts and ruptures in the larger society expose medicine to changes that will powerfully alter it.

Modern medicine shares a certain perception or view of the world and man's place in it with the other sciences. This view stresses the separation of human beings from their world and their environment. Perhaps this world view had survival value when the environment was decidedly hostile. But times have changed. We have largely subjugated Nature, although we are beginning to witness its resilience. Sustained assaults on our environment can be shown to be counterproductive. Slowly the realization is emerging that a new balance must be struck with nature if man is to survive. Whether a new balance can be struck today or whether man must further evolve in order to strike a new bargain is unanswerable.

Nevertheless, contemporary medicine is clearly and

squarely premised on the prevailing world view that separates human beings from their world. Medicine first seeks to
insulate the patient from a supposedly hostile environment,
and if that protection fails, then deploys its firepower to
destroy the hostile agent. But as we begin to discover the
interconnectedness of all of nature, and as we discover the
latent but untapped powers of human beings, we will need a
new medicine that is calibrated with what we know and can
learn. The new wisdom will stress interdependence, a merg-
ing of human beings into their environment. The new
medicine, therefore, must and will reflect new truths.

The emergence of new thinking will be slow, perhaps too
slow. But as concepts change, medicine can and must
change. Medicine was designed to deal with health, but instead it deals with disease. Health is an effect of multiple
causes, but medicine finesses nearly all the causes and treats
only the effects—the symptoms. The causes are presumably
someone else's problem. And as a result of fidelity to the
scientific model, medicine has become both microscopic and
reductionistic. It deals only with acute disease conditions and
leaves the problem of health to the patient and to the polity.
But at the same time, through professionalization and pro-
tectionism, the medical care enterprise has systematically
stripped both patient and polity of the understanding and
knowledge essential to the task.

The approach we have taken to health is limited by the
borders of our concepts; our thinking about health is limited
by the quality of our ideas. Moreover, ideas have a life span
of their own. The ideas we have about health have reached
senility. Unfortunately, the systems we fashion from our
ideas often live on long after the ideas themselves are extin-
guished. We are at that point in medicine. Where are we
going, then? Will we just play out our current ideas until our
errors are patent? Or are there some new ideas that might
animate the medicine of the future?

We are at the point of a paradigm shift in medicine. Our

perceptions of health and the systems we construct out of those perceptions are consonant with our perceptions of the world around us. If this is so, a reconstruction of where we have been and where we are should aid us in speculating about the future—a new paradigm and a new medicine.

Medicine can be said to have passed through five eras to the present. Each of these eras can be assessed in three steps: first, by characterizing the dominant world view relating to health; second, by identifying the most utilized medical technologies; and finally, by adducing the prevailing health paradigm, which can be seen as an amalgam of the world view and the technology. An analysis of these eras will generate some of the elements of a new paradigm for health in the future.

Era One: The Ages of Magic.[6] Prior to the emergence of "modern" medicine in the eighteenth century (according to some historians), medicine reflected the vicissitudes of man's relationships to the gods and to nature. Untoward events, including sickness and disease, resulted from disharmonies in these relationships. Disharmonies might arise from many causes, but chief among them was behavior offensive to the gods. These ideas appear simple, but they are rudimentary. Sickness was not an abnormal condition requiring specialized care, but was a feature of a hard existence. It resulted from imbalances in human beings' relationship to their environment.

The technology matched the rudeness of the ideas. Three elements were central. The first was the oral record. This ostensibly mythical body of tradition contained "lessons" about the healthy life. The second—rituals—sprang from the first, although repugnant curative practices (some of which were discussed earlier) were frequently incorporated. The rituals were not always arbitrary; most of them were based on empirical observations. Sacrifice was the third. This

occasionally entailed human or animal sacrifice as a means of
propitiating the gods, as, for example, in the tradition of
some Central American cultures, but more importantly
stressed self-sacrifice. Individuals or groups, presumably responsible for the affliction, subjected themselves to regimens
designed to please or pacify the authorities.

The composer, arranger, and conductor of these practices
was the shaman. The shaman is a generic historical figure in
most premodern cultures. Most shamans—again I am using
the term generically to embrace early healers from many
cultures—played two major roles. The first was to heal a
patient, and the second to heal the community. In their
healing role with patients, shamans emphasized the symbolic
aspects of healing, including the use of colorful regalia,
sacrifices, spitting of blood, and the use of fire. But since
sickness was an event that could be used to instruct the
larger community, shamans also organized cultural experiences for the community, often around the sickness of a
member. These "group healing ceremonies," as Jerome
Frank calls them, mixed curative acts, such as pulse readings, with culturally significant rituals.[7]

Too much emphasis on magic and ritual is misplaced.
Prescientific medicine, as bizarre as it often appears, was also
doggedly pragmatic. In many cases elegant rituals were
premised on sound empirical observations. Ritchie-Calder,
quoting Oliver Wendell Holmes, Sr., points out that early
medicine appropriated "everything from every source that
can be of the slightest use to anybody who is ailing in any
way."[8]

At its root, the paradigm of early medicine—the shamanistic tradition—was based on balance. Man and nature coexisted in an uneasy equilibrium that had to be restored
before individual cures and community consensus could be
achieved. Claude Lévi-Strauss characterizes the paradigm
this way:

That the mythology of the shaman does not correspond to objective reality does not matter. The patient believes in it and belongs to a society that believes in it. The protecting spirits, the evil spirits, the supernatural monsters and magical monsters are elements of a coherent system which are the basis of the natives' concept of the universe. The patient accepts them, or rather she has never doubted them. What she does not accept are the incomprehensible and arbitrary pains which represent an element foreign to her system but which the shaman, by invoking the myth, will replace in a whole in which everything has its proper place.[9]

Era Two: From Shaman to Doctor. To the shaman the body was a mysterious, almost sacred vessel. As such it was inviolate. It was also a whole. The shaman did not approach the body by breaking it into its constituent parts. But this is precisely what the doctor does; it is one of the dominant features of modern medicine. Many factors have contributed to the rise of today's medicine; the parceling of the body into pieces is only one. But it was a very important one.

The Cartesian thesis that mind and matter were divisible drove a wedge between the mind and the body that persists in medicine today despite its repudiation everywhere else. Descartes's assertion shattered the notion that man could be viewed holistically. The Cartesian division of mind and body is an overworked shibboleth. But in the intellectual history of the West it is a sharp turning point. And as a way of looking at the world, it was seized by medicine as a way of organizing its endeavor.

Prior to Descartes, medicine was a compound of magic and empirics. It relied on magical formulations, but also on techniques consistent with observations of man and nature indigenous to a given tribe or culture. But with the body freed of the larger man and conceptualized as a machine, medicine at least had a manageable subject—the metaphor of the body as a machine. The shaman was a pivotal cultural figure who utilized both healing techniques and communal ceremony. But a shaman was not needed to tinker with a machine; what was needed was a mechanic. The class of shamans could now be replaced by a class of mechanics.

Although the metaphor of man as a machine is over-worked, it is nonetheless central to an understanding of this period. As Thomas McKeown, an expert on the period, has said:

> The approach to biology and medicine established during the seventeenth century was an engineering one based on a physical model. Nature was conceived in mechanistic terms, which lead in biology to the idea that a living organism could be regarded as a machine which might be taken apart and reassembled if its structure and function were fully understood. In medicine, the same concept lead further to the belief that an understanding of disease processes and of the body's response to them would make it possible to intervene therapeutically, mainly by physical (surgical), chemical, or electrical methods.[10]

The idea of the body as a machine is elegant to the biologist and highly explanatory. However, in medicine's hands it was perverted in practice. To think of man as a machine does aid us in understanding something about bodily function and about man's role in the universe, but it does not follow that treating the body as a machine will heal it. But medicine appropriated the idea as the premise for its practice.

Just as early machines were crude, so were the early medical technologies. Medicine had largely passed beyond prescriptions based on bodily humors, but its techniques were still unsophisticated in today's terms. Bloodletting persisted, cauterization was used, and the use of purgatives was also common. But medicine remained outside the body, at least until it was clear that the body could not be understood without an examination of its inner workings any more than, today, an automobile engine can be repaired without removing the hood. The study of anatomy was about to become respectable. The first anatomy textbook was published by Vesalius in 1543. His reward was nearly universal denunciation by the church and by the academic world. It took approximately another 200 years before the investigation of what went on inside the skin was widely tolerated. And this did not occur until the metaphor of the body as a machine was firmly planted.

But despite the power of the machine image, the era was transitional. The paradigm was in flux. Antiquarian notions such as the bodily humours coexisted with observations of actual function. This was the "age of the eye," as the Renaissance has often been called. It was now expected that knowledge would be a fund of observations rather than an elaboration of theological propositions. But until Virchow's *Cellular Pathology* was published in 1858,[11] medicine remained a tentative art moving alternatively through old wisdom and new findings. The doctor had emerged, but a cohesive theoretical framework for medicine had not.

Era Three: Public Health. The first public health practitioner was the shaman, whose initiatives were crude, but pragmatic and probably effective. As an illustration, the shaman might direct that a residence contaminated by the illness of a resident be burned. Quarantine was also occasionally imposed. But these measures, while conceptually consistent with public health, were modest compared to the measures launched in the nineteenth century. As early as 1853 a physician in London, John Snow, linked a cholera epidemic to contaminated water in a public water pump. But it took the genius of Pasteur, Koch, and others, later in the century, to firmly tie infectious disease to environmental sources.[12]

Today it is common wisdom that air, water, and solid waste contain disease agents. But in the late nineteenth century the idea was startling, and ushered in an entirely new way of perceiving the environment. The medicine of the seventeenth, eighteenth, and nineteenth centuries persisted. Physicians battered patients with the old remedies; health was often the loser. The perception of man as a machine also persisted, but the breakthroughs of Pasteur and others modified the metaphor. Man was still a machine, and disease a functional disorder, but with the rise of public health it was now conceivable that defects in the machinery could be introduced by a virulent environment.

But even more important, the results were far better. Medicine had slowly improved its wares, but the health of the population had not demonstrably improved. Maternal mortality remained roughly constant, and longevity did not seem to be affected. The introduction of public health programs radically improved the health of the population. For example, Pettenkofer demonstrated that the installation of sanitary sewage systems in Munich led to immediate improvements in health status.[13] These clear and unmistakable results inevitably influenced the public's conception of health. No longer was health the result of caprice, aided by the occasionally perceptive physician. Now it was possible to engineer environmental conditions that demonstrably enhanced the opportunities for health.

The technologies of public health were more complex than those that preceded it. The physician simply needed the tools of the trade. The implementation of public health programs required larger and more complex tools. Improvements in water quality were dependent on biochemical competence, but also required political negotiations to implement, and public education to work. Nevertheless, the case was clear. Health was unquestionably improved and so public health, or population medicine, joined the physician in the pursuit of health.

The patent successes of public health forced a reconceptualization of health:

Concern for the quality of the environment achieved a rational and coherent expression during the second half of the nineteenth century. In Western Europe and then in the United States, the early phases of the Industrial Revolution had resulted in crowding, misery, accumulation of filth, horrible working and living conditions, ugliness in all the mushrooming industrial areas, and high rates of sickness and mortality everywhere. The physical and mental decadence of the working classes became intolerable to the social conscience and in addition constituted a threat to the future of industrial civilization. . . .

Our nineteenth-century forebears approached their problems through a creative philosophy of man in his environment.[14]

In other words, in the nineteenth century, a sense of health as an ecological concept emerged. To achieve health, man had to understand the delicate balance between the species and the environment. This concept was not wholly new, of course. It is a fundamental proposition of Christian theology that the earth is to serve human ends. The theories of public health fit that dominant view. In fact, we have only recently learned that as beneficial as environmental engineering has been, there can be adverse consequences. In the summer of 1974, it was discovered that antipollutant treatments of smoke and particulate matter produced through industrial activity increased the acidity level in the air on the Eastern Seaboard to potentially lethal levels. But in the nineteenth century, almost any improvement in the environment engendered an improvement in the health of the affected population. It was late in that century that man "conquered" disease. The physician had very little to contribute. The result was a paradigm of health that was nicely balanced. The environment was as amenable to engineering as the human body was to doctoring. The activities were complementary. Both the body and the environment could be treated by mechanics. There could be both patient medicine and population medicine. The marriage lasted until the early twentieth century.

Era Four: The Rise of the Sciences of Services. One of the most problematic of recent phenomena is Philippine psychic surgery. As I recounted in Chapter 3, observers of this form of practice report surgical incisions without the aid of scalpel and the expression of blood and tissue without tools.[15] Skeptical observers have also reported that seldom is the tissue and blood that of the patient undergoing treatment. This leaves one of two explanations (for practical purposes). Either the healer uses sleight of hand to express the tissue and blood, or, through means we do not understand, he "materializes" the substances. The skeptic, not accepting the possibility of materialization, then suggests that the case is one of patent fraud. This is a reasonable question, but there is a far more pertinent one: What difference does it make to the patient? Observers of psychic surgery report that it does not appear to make any difference—the outcome for the patient does not appear to depend on the transparency of the fraud.

The principal objection of modern medicine to unconventional healing is that it is fraudulent, that it fails to utilize accepted tools and techniques, in short that it is "unscientific." The result is that the battle between modern medicine and other healing therapies is joined on the wrong question. The question of the impact on the patient is not raised—but it is the crucial question. One of the reasons that the question is not asked is that the answer is potentially embarrassing. Few procedures and processes used in modern medicine can be correlated with a beneficial outcome to the patient.[16] To repeat, patients can be cured by contemporary allopathic medicine and by practices like psychic surgery, but there is little more hard evidence that the technologies used in contemporary medicine have anything more to do with the outcome to the patient than those utilized in psychic surgery. This is not to say that fraud is widespread in today's medicine, but rather to say that the question of fraud is irrelevant, if a healthy outcome to a patient is the concern.

The rejection of nonallopathic healing is premised on its lack of a scientific base.[17] But medicine, in rejecting unscientific practices, acts like the reformed alcoholic: it has not had a scientific base for more than a few decades.

During the flowering of public health in the nineteenth century, the practice of medicine was also undergoing a transformation. In 1856 Claude Bernard published *An Introduction to the Study of Experimental Medicine.*[18] Bernard's book was an attack on the concept of "vitalism" in medicine—that there was a vital force which, although not understood, was responsible for health and well-being.[19] Bernard believed that events had causes, and that phenomena occurred as the result of discernible "laws."

The pursuit of laws that govern human functioning persists today. But medicine did not fully adopt a scientific approach until early this century; and even here, there is continuity. The image of man as a machine was not lost, the machine was simply recognized as a more complex instrument. The idea that contributed to the view of the world which guided medicine was repeatability, the notion that a given medical intervention would produce the same result in every patient, controlling, of course, for some individual differences, including age and fitness. The results of medical care then were not idiosyncratic. There were patterns that could be predicted because the results of care followed logically from the choice of intervention. The hypothesis was the diagnosis, the experiment was the intervention, and the confirmation was the cure. Medicine had finally left the world of magic; what was now important was the refinement of technique. If the results of care were dependent on specified interventions, then what was important was the precision of the techniques—the more precision, the more accurate the prediction, and the more the results were repeatable.

The technologies of scientific medicine were aimed at reducing the tolerance for error. The patient was a machine and would necessarily respond to carefully programmed interventions. Hence, the hospital was necessary to immobilize the patient in need of the more radical interventions, featuring surgery and chemotherapy. If patients in need of specified techniques could be placed into a homogenous environment, fewer variables could influence the result. But the physician could also influence the result if he modified the rules of the game. Technicians were needed because fine tooling was needed; artists were unwelcome. In 1910, as a result of the Flexner report,[20] the supply of medical schools was reduced to those most capable of turning out finely trained clinicians—the first of a technical class of healers. This, then, is the period when medicine indisputably shifted its focus from the anthropological to the technical.

A related technology was the measurement of health. Even the eighteenth century physicians were fascinated with the taxonomy of disease. In the nineteenth century it became an obsession. Measurement was integral to technical medicine. If machine tooling was the task, machine tolerances required computation. The classification of disease was equally important. Disease conditions had to be placed into categories so that appropriate techniques could be utilized according to the category into which the patient was placed.

But the flowering of the technology was the service system. Prior to the twentieth century, patients pursued cures. But at the turn of the century more was needed. Health could now be conceptualized as a commodity, a product that could be delivered over and over again if enough variables could be controlled. Hence, a delivery system was needed to facilitate the smooth delivery of the product. A need was perceived—patients with specific diseases. A product was conceptualized to meet the need—medical care services. Product differentiation produced an array of services, including surgery, drugs, and diagnostic tools. Distribution could be handled through hospitals and physicians' offices, which would be linked together by the physician gaining the privileges of hospital practice. And finally, marketing and promotion would be entrusted to insurance companies, largely controlled by physicians and ultimately by governmental underwriting.

The delivery system was born in this era but its maturation was a few decades away. The concept of a delivery system —an amalgam of emerging technologies—was consistent with the health paradigm of the period. Disease was a malfunction in the human machine, caused either by an internal disorder, or by the activity of an external agent. The most effective way to treat disease was first to accurately classify it, then to apply to it a set of techniques designed to produce a like cure in like patients. Since what was to be done was deliver a service, increasingly thought of as a commodity, a delivery system was created. It was in this period that medicine became almost entirely disease-oriented. And it was also this period that witnessed the rise of technical medicine, and the attrition of the arts of medicine. Medicine was close to being synonymous with health.

Era Five: The Medicine of Today. Much of this book is devoted to the description and analysis of modern medicine. Chapter 3, for example, contains a fairly detailed treatment of the delivery system. Most of these points do not need to be repeated. The purpose of this section is to isolate those characteristics of modern medicine that underpin the current medical paradigm.

Our view of health is about the same as it was in the early part of this century. Disease is still presumed to be the result of faulty machinery. And because all machines are roughly the same, treatments are finely tuned to fit discrete diagnoses.

But things have become more refined. Specialization is inexorable, and the delivery system has become so highly elaborated that the average patient is often greatly confused. But most significant has been the further conceptualization of the patient as a machine of great complexity. In the past physicians may have thought of their patients as machines, but nevertheless had to treat them as whole machines. Today, with the exception of a few hardy rural practitioners and family physicians, medicine has compartmentalized the body into finer and finer machine parts. It is one thing to treat a patient as a machine, ignoring a rich store of information that is related to health and functioning, and yet another to further subdivide the machine into its constituent parts. In the former medicine, at least the possibility existed for holistic treatment. In today's medicine the task is nearly impossible.

The technologies of today's medicine reflect its imperviousness to factors conducive to health. Surgery has become more prevalent and more profound. Drugs flow nearly unimpeded from doctor to patient, and are often prescribed for conditions like viral disorders, for which there is no chemical cure. The delivery system has become large, unwieldy, and complex—an industry in search of newer and refined products. Some of the more elaborate technologies illustrate the preoccupation of the system with technical engineering. The coronary care unit and the kidney dialysis machine link the patient, the machine, into a fixed feedback loop with another machine.

Modern medicine is only one approach to health—a wholly disease-oriented approach. Its paradigm of healing assumes that highly refined techniques and profound interventions into the body can produce health by eliminating the

symptoms of disease. This has led to the neglect of population medicine because there is no paying consumer; the
neglect of social and environmental conditions, because
physicians are only trained to intervene at the individual
level; the neglect of a blizzard of phenomena about the
human being, because it does not fit the paradigm; and
finally neglect of the role of the individual in achieving
health, because if health is a commodity it must be delivered
to a manipulable public.

The conclusion that modern medicine is disease-oriented
is easy to reach. Take the hospital. The purpose of a hospital
is to classify, confine, and immobilize. Admission is contin-
gent on appropriate classification of a disease condition. The
patient is then confined in quarters that are much the same
everywhere. This is because to the physician the human
being is simply a machine with interchangeable parts. A
given disease can be treated identically in Peoria or in
Phoenix; it is the disease that is being treated, not the person. This also accounts for the immobilization of the patient.
Aside from its convenience to the harried doctor, immobilization is the same as turning off the engine in a car and
leaving it in a stall at the mechanic's shop. The car and the
human are both machines in need of repair.

But there is more to it. While we do not know enough
about what produces health we know some things—com-
monsense things. For example, we know that a nutritious
diet, recreation, fresh air, and sunlight are related to health.
But because the hospital is a factory for the repair of disease,
none of these things are readily available. Hospital food is
not only tasteless, it is not nutritious—nothing is fresh,
everything is frozen, white bread and butter are served, and
so on. There is no opportunity for recreation and exercise in
a hospital. There could be gyms and exercise rooms, but a
person doing yoga or any other bodily exercise faces deri-
sion, even prohibition. And there is little opportunity to be

outdoors; hospitals are hermetically sealed chambers. The only way a patient can get outdoors (if there are any grounds) is to grope his or her way to the front door and then face the possibility of alarm from the matrons at the admissions desk.

The modern hospital is one of the unhealthiest places around.

Today's medicine has succeeded where the medicines of the past have failed: it has succeeded in equating medical care with health. But the borders of the paradigm are blurring. It is becoming increasingly clear that health is not the same as medicine. The wrong questions have deservedly received the wrong answers. A new paradigm for health is slowly emerging.

A NEW PARADIGM

The history of health has been the history of adaptation. Through biological adaptation man has survived; and through adaptation, not medical care, man has achieved improved health. Today, postindustrial man faces a new set of challenges to adaptation. The environmental insults of the industrial age—contaminated water and lack of sanitation, the unavailability of basic nutrients, uncontrolled epidemics and an inadequate understanding of infectious transmission—have been mostly managed. But the insults of today have not. These include air quality, chemical treatments of foodstuffs and other products, overindulgence in food and drugs, stress, the pace of life, congestion, noise, and the lack of recreation and exercise. The contribution of medical care was minor in the adaptation of man to the industrial threats to health; and similarly, it has only a minor role to play in the adaptations that now face us. The reason lies in the paradigm of health that medicine has conceived—the "science of the organized individual," to use A. C. Crombie's term. Crombie elaborates:

> The biology of the individual is more like engineering than physics, in that each type of living organism is a solution to a specific set of engineering problems—problems of intake and conversion of fuel, locomotion, communication, replication and so on which it has to solve to survive. This subject matter has imposed on physiology its characteristic program: to find out how an organism works by taking it to pieces and trying to put it together again from knowledge of the parts.[21]

Medicine has ignored the understanding of man that is implicit in evolutionary theory, historical demography, and medical ecology. As a result it has sought to engineer human health through the manipulation of human parts. John Powles has examined this question in some detail in his paper "On the Limitations of Modern Medicine":

> The engineering approach to the improvement of health has been dominant over an alternative approach which would emphasize the importance of way of life factors in disease—an approach which could be described as "ecological." While it is to changes with which the latter is concerned that industrial man largely owes his current standard of health, it is in the engineering approach that he has placed his faith. Curative medicine has not been very successful in reducing the impact of diseases of maladaptation.[22]

To Powles, as to me, the problem is that,

> Enthusiasm for the system has outpaced its concrete achievements and its indirect costs tend to be underplayed. Despite the evidence to the contrary, it is widely believed by both patients and their doctors that industrial populations owe their high health standards to "scientific medicine," that such medical technology as currently exists is largely effective in coping with the tasks it faces and that it offers great promise for the future.[23]

Tolstoy, in a quote used by Powles, captures the mood of medicine perfectly in "The Death of Ivan Illyich":

> The doctor said: this-and-that indicates that this-and-that is wrong with you, but if an analysis of this-and-that does not confirm our diagnosis, we must suspect you of having this-and-that. If we assume that you have this-and-that, then . . . and so on. There was only one question Ivan Illyich wanted answered: was his condition dangerous or not? But the doctor ignored that question as irrelevant. From the doctor's point of view, such a question was unworthy of consideration. One had only to weigh possibilities: floating kidneys, chronic catarrh, or an ailment of the caecum. There was no question of the life of Ivan Illyich—nothing but a contest between floating kidneys and the caecum. In the presence of Ivan Illyich the doctor gave a brilliant solution to the problem in favour of the caecum, with the reservation that the analysis of his water might supply new information necessitating a reconsideration of the case.[24]

Something different is needed. The medicine of today pits man against a hostile world. But it is in the relationship between human beings and their environment that the key to health lies. Health then is not just the well-oiled functioning of the body—it is achieved through the strategic collaboration of human beings with their world expressed through a series of "relationships." These include the relationship between mind and matter; humans and nature; humans and the social roles they play; and humans and higher consciousness, even spirituality. The physician can help, but the individual must be responsible for those relationships. It is individuals who must "learn" to control bodily processes, including those heretofore considered involuntary. It is individuals who must relearn their interconnectedness with nature. And it is individuals who must discover their higher, more spiritual, capacities by expanding their consciousness and self-awareness.

This may sound utopian but it is, in most respects, where we started.

THE OBSTACLES

There will be resistance to sweeping change. When even modest reform is difficult, revolution may appear to be romantic escapism. But though a revolution is necessary, it need not be bloody. If the moral and conceptual underpinning under medicine erodes, as I have suggested it will, the revolution in medicine will be bloodless because it will take place at the level of concepts. But since shifts in values and attitudes often occur slowly, something dramatic is needed now. Medicine is failing us now. Moreover, inescapable pressures are mounting for reform of the system within conventional bounds. Consequently, unless revolutionary concepts can be formulated out of which new approaches grow, the changes that will occur will strengthen the existing delivery system. What is needed is a shift in paradigms, not organizational and financing reforms. Health is not a commodity for packaging, seller to buyer, but a rich web of causes, effects, and interactions. Resources play a part, as does social and environmental engineering; but individuals must also integrate their own knowledge with the use of healers.

Underlying these reforms is the need for a radical reconceptualization of health and behavior related to health. The most fundamental message of this book is that no amount of social and systems engineering will replace the need to think differently about health.

Even given fresh, lively ideas, the pursuit of health will not be an easy task. Institutional reforms and attitudinal changes are hard to accomplish. There are many obstacles. Chief among them is the institutional pressures of medicine in the United States. It is the largest social service system in the world, and it employs more people than any other sector of the economy, with the exception of education. Any proposal to reduce the size of the system will necessarily meet strong resistance. Other problems include the lack of a coherent policy for the aged, the value preferences of an indulged public that chooses chewing gum, sugar, fatty foods, high-speed cars, and spectator sports; and the power of industries that market the products that a complacent, ignorant public consumes.

These constraints are formidable; they deserve more attention. Since resistance will be fierce, some of the specific objections can be anticipated.

The Radical Critique.   Not unlike the boy who cried wolf, the conventional assaults on profits and exploitation of the consumer in the medical establishment are wearing thin. They are accurate, but shortsighted. The wrong targets have been chosen, and the clamor has excited a backlash. Medicine continues to be beleaguered from many sides, but some apologists are showing up. In *The Case for American Medicine,*[25] Harry Schwartz typifies the response to the radical assault. He reluctantly acknowledges the infirmities such as maldistribution, high costs, and barriers to access, but argues that the solution lies neither in reform nor in revolution, but rather in the installation of incentives to stimulate structural refinements within the system.

Schwartz is shrill in his own fashion—particularly when railing against health maintenance organizations (HMO's), the newly established prepaid medical care outfits.[26] But his analysis is systemic—he proposes changes within the existing system. He differs little in analytic terms from the radical reformers who also desire systemic change, albeit more sweeping. For example, Schwartz pines for the bygone days of the dedicated practitioner, dispensing homely wisdom along with an occasional swift and sudden cure. Even the AMA has abandoned this barricade.

In *The American Health Empire: Power, Profits and Politics,*[27] the authors, members of the Health Policy Advisory Center (Health-PAC), seem to share Schwartz's sympathy for the rude past:

The health industry has come a long way from the days of the one-horse patent medicine peddler with his line of liver pills and elixirs. Replacing him are the mammoth internationalist drug companies, whose corporate medicine chests are increasingly likely to include hospital supplies, computers, and cosmetics along with a growing profusion of pills. Health insurance, which can trace its origins to pretrade union workers' welfare funds, is now a key element of the nation's vast insurance industry. The hospital supply industry has outgrown its bandaid days and is branching into catheters, computers, and artificial organs. Proprietaries, which used to be the dark horse of the delivery system, are forging multistate chains and moving into more and more investors' portfolios.[28]

Where Schwartz (and other apologists) and the radicals part is on politics. Schwartz wants society to stay where it is. Conversely, the radicals desire to powerfully transform society along equalitarian lines. Medicine is a part of this struggle. If the analyst does not want society to change, then it follows that medicine cannot roil the waters. But if society is to move, then medicine must also move, because it is intimately linked with the social structure.

This book parts company from both camps. In Chapter 3, the "system" was explored, but in hoary clichés, because the ground has been so trampled that little original can be said. I agree with the radical critique, as far as it goes, except for one thing. It insists on widening and deepening access to care when the counterintuitive nature of that step can be demonstrated. I am not saying that there are not unmet health needs, especially among the poor, which must first be met in any transformation of the system. But that fact should not be used as an argument to deter the needed transformation.

I have little sympathy for the apologist. The system is a perversion, an almost ridiculous example of the penchant of governments, particularly in the United States, to trade off human lives for "immutable" principles. But both armies —the radicals and the apologists—are skirmishing in the wrong field. The war will be fought elsewhere, where transformations in society take place that transcend politics, and clearly transcend "health politics."

The Scientific Critique. Next are objections to my central thesis. What about arguments that medicine is more highly related to health than I have argued and that, contrary to my expectations, medicine's role will and must grow rather than diminish?

In a recent *Los Angeles Times* article, Dr. Alex Gerber, a clinical professor of medicine at the University of Southern California, advanced the stock argument. The crisis in medical care, he argued, is a crisis of demand and supply. In brief, our health care problems can be solved only with a massive infusion of new physicians. Dr. Gerber asserts that "evidence of physician shortages is all around us. . . . [D]espite medical advances, the thrust for medical personnel and facilities remains unabated and often increases."[29]

The proposal offered by Dr. Gerber, which is consistent with the AMA's position, is premised on two points. First, that the solution to the crisis in medical care is more of the same. This is the antithesis of my argument. Not only will more of the same fail to improve health, the costs will be staggering, and the net impact may even be a loss of health. As Dr. Gerber points out, with current dollars it costs about $100,000 to train a physician. And 22,000 new physicians will be needed each year on the basis of his projections. That amounts to an outlay of more than $2 billion per year in new costs just for physician manpower. The fact that the availability of physicians has not been shown to correlate with health does not seem to disturb him.

Recent experience in the United Kingdom is also pertinent. When the National Health Service was founded the assumption was that costs would be brought under control. The reasoning was that unmet health needs would be met and expected improvements in health status would dampen demand. But costs have not been controlled; on the contrary, they have sharply and steadily risen. And the major reason is that health status has *not* improved, nor will it if health is thought of as the consequent of medical care services.

The second argument Dr. Gerber raises (and only by implication) is much less tractable. Most apologists for the current system argue that more supply—more doctors and hospital beds—is needed because the demand is so intense; many towns have no doctors, and so on. There is a double-edged irony here. First, it is true that there is demand, occasionally shrill. But much of that demand has been stimulated by providers. It is the provider who decides whether there is a health problem, how much it will cost to fix it, and how long it will last. Second, it is that very demand, triggered and nourished by the provider, that results in profound dependency on services. The provider points to demand as the excuse for augmenting supply. But this is disingenuous. A large portion of the demand for health services is an artifact. And because the demand is pressed by helpless consumers, its existence is testimony to the failure of medicine to engender health habits. It is the most feudal aspect of medicine.

But the fact remains that people demand medical care, not health. Rashi Fein, a Harvard-based economist, perceptively characterizes consumer demand as a, if not the, major obstacle to reform. Fein acknowledges the validity of my central thesis, but then points out that:

> In the case of health and medical care, we are dealing with a sector in which, because of customs and folkways, image may be even more important than reality. Because some (even if relatively little) medical care deals with matters of life and death, because of fear, because of infatuation with science and technology—as well as because medicine oftentimes does help some individuals and, therefore, each individual can hope that

it will help him—persons have come to believe that medical
care services and intervention by the physician make significant
contributions to health. This view is not likely to change.[30]

It is a hard point. I agree that consumer demand for individual treatment frustrates new approaches. But I have
not argued that the revolution can be accomplished in six
days with a day of rest. It will take a long time. And the
hardest task will be education. And medicine will oppose the
changes I propose. Correctional personnel often oppose
prison reform, and many lawyers oppose no-fault automobile compensation.

Others will argue that I have overstated the case. Perhaps
I have. Medicine can and does cure. All I have said is that it
cures far less than is generally understood and that its modalities of treatment, whether effective or not, can cause
more ill health than is cured. Moreover, I have argued that
medicine must be placed in a broader context so that comparisons can be made between its impact on health with
other factors, social, environmental, and personal. In es-
sence, then, aside from the need for new ideas, all that I
have argued, peeled to its core, is that the size, scope, and
cost of medicine be reduced and calibrated with its relative
influence on the ultimate goal—healthy individuals and a
healthy population.

And finally, to those who argue that, even if what I have
said about medicine's impact on health is accurate, the "end
of medicine" is unlikely because it is too deeply a part of our
culture, and that the arguments I have offered about a
widespread sociocultural transformation are unconvincing,
all I can say is to look around you again, and if you still are
not convinced, wait a year and then look again.

The "People Won't Change" Critique.   Another serious charge
is that people do not want to be healthy. This is probably

true. We do not know much about healthy behaviors, and most of us ignore what we do know. In a major study of 62 smoking control programs, Jerome Schwartz concluded that most failed because of dropout.[31] But even for those who desire to live healthy lives, the task is hard. We are exposed to smoke wherever we go; air quality is beyond our control except in the most indirect way; hours and style of work are often inflexible; traffic congestion and associated stress is inescapable for most; and many do not know enough to eat well, even if they can afford to do so.

But there is some hope. People cannot be compelled to be healthy, but opportunities can be enhanced—health education, expanded recreation, staggered working days, and so on, are possibilities. Attitudinal change is also possible; smoking has decreased, presumably as the result of information. It takes time, but gradually the implications should seep in. Finally, interventions into the environment can be made that benefit everyone without the need for individual compliance. For example, if the safeguards on nuclear power plant emissions are effective, the health of everyone potentially exposed is assured, even though no individual act is required by those who benefit.

There is a danger here though—individual freedoms must be preserved. Imprisonment for political sabotage is not significantly different from imprisonment for failure to jog six miles a week. A health czar is not what we need. But some prohibitions might be acceptable—for example, on smoking in public places—if made through democratic and participatory means.

The danger is a serious one. The medicine I have argued for in this book presupposes that society place a high value on health. If the threshold conditions for health are to be raised, and if people are to be encouraged to alter their life styles, health must be more highly prized. In part this will only happen if people experience the difference in their lives that full health brings. And in part it can only happen if the public can be persuaded to limit their use of medical care to liberate the resources needed to pursue health. But there is still the threat to individual freedoms. If people wish to destroy their health, should they not be allowed to do so? Incentives to health might be offered. If people want to ride motorcycles without wearing helmets and so bust their heads open, that's OK, but society need not necessarily subsidize such adventures by paying for the medical care costs to patch them up. But even if this were a plausible policy, it is still doubtful that people can be forced to be healthy. Consequently, until and unless society places a higher value on health, we will be less healthy than we could be *and* we will be stuck with the medicine we have because we neither can afford a new medicine, nor tolerate a medicine that promotes health rather than repairs the sick.[32] This may seem an unlikely development, but much of what I have offered in this book is an argument that it can happen. We are on a high-technology–low-humanism trajectory in health, but a shift is possible—a shift to a medicine with low technology and high humanism.

The "Practical" Critique. Finally, there is the argument that the proposals are hopelessly utopian; they are overstated, and they fail to reflect an understanding of how change occurs. The argument can be broken into four parts: first, allegations that there is too much stress on individual responsibility, particularly since we know so little about disease; second, that the elimination of barriers to practice will result in charlatanism and quackery; third, that change will not occur without an appropriate strategy or game plan featuring incremental steps and the use of incentives; and fourth and finally, that the changes proposed are impossible because they are too expensive.

I have stressed the role of the individual; I have even argued that it is paramount. I have done so for two reasons.

First, modern medicine has emasculated the patient. The patient is given little opportunity to participate in his or her illness. Most of us panic at the onset of illness; our invariable reaction is to summon a physician and then give up. This places far too much stress on the healer and the therapy. I have stressed the individual's role in an effort to restore the individual's proper role in health and "healthing." Although there are instances when the individual truly heals without help, unquestionably there are other instances when help is needed and should be sought. I have not argued that the individual must lie on a procrustean bed of illness and fight on alone. Medical care should be available, and there should be people who care, especially for those who have no relatives and friends. But a balance must be struck, and in my view the scale is far too heavily weighted on the side of the healer. The healer should do what is possible when aid is sought, but the individual must assume the ultimate responsibility for his or her health. To do otherwise is to expect too much of the healer.

The second reason can be more simply stated, and perhaps is more important. I have stressed the individual role because, based on everything I have come across in the preparation of this book, the responsible individual is clearly the most important factor in achieving health. This is a bold assertion. However, my conclusion has some support. Certainly Jerome Frank's work, to which I have repeatedly referred, is essentially in support. But another example can be found in the work of Lester Breslow and his colleagues, who surveyed the health behavior of about 7000 Californians for five and a half years. Although it is true that Californians may not be a representative sample (for health habits or anything else), the investigators established strong links between health habits, including regular sleep, weight maintenance, smoking and alcohol consumption, and exercise and health. None of this is very shocking, but the importance of the research is that adherence to health habits are the responsibility of the individual. As Breslow concludes, "We are reaching the point where *individual responsibility* is a highly important factor in determining good health."[33]

The second "practical" objection arises from a concern that quackery is sure to result if the system is deprofessionalized. I have suggested that the professional stranglehold on the provision of services and health information be broken.[34] There are some dangers. But since so many of the other reforms will founder unless professionalism is eroded, it is necessary to do so. There will be some quackery; it is unavoidable where money is to be made out of human suffering. But there are two serious arguments. First, as I have said, we do not know much about what heals and what does not. As conventional research is conducted, we discover what conventionally works. But we also know that there are less conventional factors at work, factors that are unlikely to be assessed, or in some cases allowed into the healing equation in the first place. Some of these are the scale of the facility in which care is rendered; the nature and behavior of health personnel; the setting for care—home, outpatient, hospital; the powers of healing of those who claim to be healers; and the role of the family and of the patient. Unless the barriers to practice are lowered to allow the interplay of new mixtures of personnel and facilities and interpersonal interactions, these factors are unlikely to be fully assessed.

The second argument is closely related to the first. The theories and practices on which contemporary medicine is premised are not the only ones. There are other theories and other medical practices. And there is evidence, some of which has been discussed, that these systems of medicine are effective. The rigorous professionalization of modern medicine has succeeded in barring, or at least constraining practitioners employing alternative therapies and techniques, such as acupuncture and chiropractic. The opportunity to learn from alternative practices should not be lost, but will be if the prevailing barriers to practice remain. One example: Sister Justa Smith, a biochemist, has isolated a factor that may be associated with healing. Since her hypothesis is that enzyme activity is related to the healing process, she examined persons who claimed to be healers to determine whether they could accelerate enzyme activity. Her research thus far is confirmatory. Some of those who claim to be healers and appear to have had success in healing can dramatically elevate enzyme activity in controlled experiments.[35] If this is so, although much more research needs to be done, why should the natural healer be a hunted species?

Quackery will occur but can be dealt with in three ways. First, as information becomes available linking the processes of care with patient outcomes, information will be available to aid people in making choices about healers. Second, that same information will make it possible to bar some practitioners from practice at regional health centers, when it is clear that harm is being done to patients. Third, communities may also choose to bar some practitioners from association with neighborhood hospitals.

The rapidity and scale of change is the focus of the third objection. The argument is that the reforms I propose are hopelessly unrealistic because they are inconsistent with prevailing social, political, and economic realities. In addition, it is argued that since some of the proposals have merit, they might be achieved step by step, particularly if appropriate incentives to change are utilized. It is true that change occurs in this gradualist way, and some proposals, such as the regionalization of costly medical care equipment and services, could be implemented without a titanic struggle. But if the reforms I propose are viewed as a whole, the conclusion is inescapable—a revolution is needed. As I have said, the revolution must occur at the level of concepts. If we start to think differently about health, the reforms will follow in due course.

In a brilliant paper, "Hierarchical Restructuring," John Platt, a futurologist and biophysicist, characterizes the nature of rapid change in the structure of systems.[36] The examples include the Industrial Revolution, the French Revolution, and the design and construction of the U.S. Constitution. Platt points to five characteristics of rapid system change:

1. The accumulation of "bits" of data that do not fit the old predictions, or old explanations.
2. The fact that the change is preceded by widespread dissonance and is followed, when the transformation takes place, by widespread change.
3. The change is very sudden and is consummated in a relatively short period of time, contrasted with the "life" of the system which is replaced.
4. The change is often in the direction of "simplification"; more simple explanations and practices.
5. Finally, and more subtle, is the occurrence of interactions "leaping" across the system level between the old system and the new system in the process of formation, which precede the transformation.

This analysis fits my analysis. It is far from self-evident that medicine will change dramatically in the next few years, but there are enough signs and signals to make it a possibility.

Finally, it will be argued that insufficient resources would be saved from the truncation of the existing medical care system to establish the programs that are proposed. This may be true in the initial conversion of the system because of pending commitments and sunk costs, and because existing needs must be met before the long-range benefits of the new programs are experienced. But we must bite the bullet sometime. If prevention works, the demands on a frozen and partially retreaded personal health care system will gradually lessen, permitting reallocation of resources to new programs until some reasonable equilibrium is reached.

It will also be argued that we will have enough revenue to preserve medicine and launch new programs as well. I do not agree. The press of existing social and domestic needs is so great that substantially more money will be demanded. Medicare is not the only claimant. There are limits to public expenditures. Health care resources for the aged population alone in 2000 will be enormous. The current system is likely to consume 10 percent or more of the gross national product by the year 2000. But even assuming that sufficient monies could be commandeered, why should the existing system be preserved at the expense of amelioration of other problems? As Ivan Illich has said:

> Each car which Brazil puts on the road denies fifty people good transportation by bus. Each merchandized refrigerator reduces the chance of building a community freezer. Every dollar spent in Latin America on doctors and hospitals costs a hundred lives. . . . Had each dollar been spent on providing safe drinking water, a hundred lives could have been saved.[37]

Things are not so different here.

Health and National Health Insurance: The Counter-Intuitive Program. In the face of sharp criticism of medical care, a solution to the ills of the system is now being sought through the enactment of a national health insurance program. Bills have been introduced by the American Medical Association, Senators Long and Ribicoff, the National Health Insurance Association of America, the Nixon Administration, Senator Edward Kennedy on behalf of the Committee of One Hundred and the AFL-CIO, UAW, and other labor groups, and the American Hospital Association. Enactment of a national health insurance plan in the United States can probably be expected within the next few years.

Although the plans differ in their approaches to the means of financing care, the total number of federal and state dollars to be appropriated, and the nature and degree of public regulation, they all have three things in common. First, all tend to build upon the existing delivery system, although many of the plans propose further industrialization of the system. Second, they share a failure to address a major alternative to the existing delivery system—a national health service—along the lines of the medical care systems in Great Britain and Sweden and some other Western nations. And third, there is no recognition of the limitations of medical care to engender health.

Fidelity to the existing system is expected. The existing system has an effective lobby. But alternatives have not been cogently and forcefully offered. And, irrespective of the arguments for and against a national health service—the second of the points—its viability in the United States is doubtful.

The reason why there has been no debate about the third point—the limits of medicine—must be sought outside the policy-making process. Observers and practitioners of medical care have failed to grasp the implications of the evidence. It is difficult to acknowledge that what we are doing is not working. And it is extremely difficult to pose alternatives. As a result, the burning issue of the day is national health insurance, not the end of medicine.

One virtue we have been consistently willing to compromise is egalitarianism. We have tolerated tiers of medical practice paralleling class structure and even have created classes of medical untouchables. Medicare and Medicaid have reduced some of these distinctions. Their logical extension has always been some form of comprehensive national health insurance that would greatly expand public support of medical care while leaving the delivery system intact.

National health insurance was a major issue in the 1972 presidential election, and the debate has continued in Congress since then. Thus, the assault proposed against inequitable access to care in this country will be made with dollars rather than with structural reform. The solution being advanced, despite differences in details, is to increase purchasing power to a level that presumably would be relatively uniform throughout the population. But those with expanded purchasing power will be buying more of the same. This indictment applies to all of the major national health insurance proposals, including the polar approaches espoused by Senator Kennedy and the AMA. To be sure, there are differences of real substance in the pending proposals. But when measured against the arguments made here, the plans are all of a piece. The current debate is proceeding along a narrow track. Nowhere does one hear discussion of the issues I have raised. And failure to engage these issues will have two profound and irreversible consequences.

The first is that major expansion in the financing system will lock in the current system for delivery of care for the indefinite future. This is the pitfall of the otherwise salutary means being taken to assault inequities in medical care through an expansion of purchasing power. The issue must be so stated as to make it possible for those who wish to limit the scope of the existing system to fix on that goal and not be deflected by the benefits that comprehensive health insurance will ostensibly provide.

The second is that underwriting the costs of medical care through a comprehensive health insurance plan will inevitably result in even steeper escalations in the cost of care and a more disproportionate consumption of the gross national product by medical care. Enoch Powell, based on his years of experience in administering England's health service (and leaving aside his animadversions on other subjects), has marveled at the capacity of patients to consume large doses of care. The passage of a national health insurance plan will dissolve the last consumption constraint—the lack of uniform purchasing power. As a nation we will have then decided to further feed an already bloated system and in so doing divert monies that could otherwise be spent to ameliorate social and environmental conditions that have a demonstrably greater impact on health, such as poor housing and malnutrition. And, most tragically, we will deepen the dependency of consumers on services and providers.

Because we are on the verge of putting public monies to the task that private money and health care professionals have not accomplished, the prospects for a new medicine are dim. Thus, passage of a national health insurance plan poses a real and poignant conflict to those who wish to devise and implement a system of medical care that will deal with causes, not cures, and with health rather than disease. The failure to promote a new medicine means that "the future belongs to illness," to use Peter Sedgewick's phrase:

> we just are going to get more and more diseases, since our expectations of health are going to become more expansive and sophisticated. Maybe one day there will be a backlash, perhaps at the point where everybody has become so luxuriantly ill. . . . [B]ut for the moment, it seems that illness is going to be "in"; a rising tide of really chronic sickness.[38]

Health and Well-Being.   The end of medicine is not the end of health but the beginning. To achieve health, we must enlarge freedom from material want. Of course, the opportunity to seek well-being is not widespread, but the resources are available and could be tapped if they were not harnessed to the causes of war, competition, and exploitation. And those uses and misuses of our resources must come to an end as well, if not through revolution then at least through natural attrition and decay.

We must also achieve a change at the conceptual level. We have neither sought health nor revered the healthy individual. We have failed to do so because we have not understood what health is—we have been confused by an assumption that it was an alloy of good luck and medical care. But in the next few decades our understanding will deepen. The pursuit of health and of well-being will then be possible, but only if our environment is made safe for us to live in and our social order is transformed to foster health, rather than suppress joy. If not, we shall remain a sick and dependent people. In this sense, Virchow was profoundly right: Medicine is simply a form of politics.

Epilogue

A Design for
the Future

This epilogue contains some of my personal views about the medicine of the future. Starting over, even conceptually, is an extremely difficult task. We do know, in broad terms, what is likely to be more effective, but we do not know enough. But there are some basic points:

1. We must vastly expand programs of health education. People must be given the opportunity to gain a greater understanding of their bodies, of the signals they receive. We must also teach people to help one another. As simple and even conventional as this sounds, it is unquestionably the most important step. But it should also be understood that I am not proposing third-grade classes in personal hygiene. Health education should be far more sophisticated than that; there is more to health than brushing one's teeth every day. Health education should be a major component in any curriculum, particularly during the adolescent years when health habits are developed. The task is a large one; the knowledge deficit is great and will take time to overcome.

Health education should also be available in hospitals. Almost every hospital has some space that could be made available for community health education programs. Among other things, films, seminars, lectures, and meetings could be sponsored. Both written and graphic materials could be made available. And some of the tools of care, such as bandages, splints, and some medications, could be explained and distributed. To fund these programs initially, all hospitals in receipt of federal assistance could be required to make space and resources available.

2. We need substantially more information about health behaviors. Our science focuses on what agents cause disease, *not* on what interactions introduce and maintain health. We recognize the influence of diet and nutrition and the benefits of exercise, even if we do not know exactly how they benefit us. But we have not learned how to motivate people to take more responsibility for themselves and to adopt healthy behaviors. In short, we need research trained on the healthy and their behaviors. The only evidence we have now is the occasional anecdote about the 136-year-old Bolivian peasant who attributes his longevity to liquor and loose women.

3. The existing system should be rigorously deprofessionalized. Certification should be substituted for current licensure schemes. The system would require that the healer give full notification to prospective patients of his or her training, if any, and treatment modalities utilized, costs, and so on. This certification system should be coupled with publication of the outcomes of therapy by individual healers and health care institutions.[1]

4. We will still need services, treatments, and cures. Medical care can cure; what works should be preserved. Nonetheless, the current system must be diminished to about half its current size. In countries that have medical care systems much smaller than ours, health is not measurably worse than in the United States.

5. One element that should be preserved, because it works, is the care and treatment of the acutely ill. Physicians should practice directly with and in acute care facilities, which in most cases will be existing hospitals, when the hospital has the capacity to provide such care. Acute care facilities should also develop greatly improved emergency

care facilities. Expenditures for acute care should be determined on a cost-effective basis. Budgetary requests should compete for the available dollars with other programs.

6. Physicians, other than those involved in acute and emergency care, should be redeployed and retrained, if necessary, to design and staff the prevention programs outlined below. They should be allowed to treat patients with conditions not requiring hospitalization in acute care facilities only through or in connection with prevention programs, or in residential complexes for the aged. For those practitioners who cannot be retrained, or who cannot find positions, jobs should be offered in any areas that continue to be underserved. The remainder will have to join the ranks of the technologically unemployed.

7. New or retrained health personnel will be needed. For example, persons might be trained to provide initial detection and diagnostic services and some limited treatment for ambulatory patients. Also, persons should be trained to provide initial screening and nonacute remedial services to persons residing in areas currently without such services. Such new personnel should be trained in medical schools until such time as the faculty and administrative staff of such schools can be pared to the size appropriate to train the lesser number of fully-trained physicians required, or redeployed to train an array of healers. Over the next 10 years or so, health sciences programs should be totally redesigned to train health personnel along a continuum of need, with the acute care physician at one pole.

8. Drugs, once checked for efficacy, should be made available for purchase by patients without a prescription, along with a complete and intelligible description of the drug, its appropriate use, and potential side effects. Similarly, many of the simple tools of medical care—bandages, splints, clamps, and some simple surgical tools—should be made available for general use.

9. A special need will exist for the training of persons in

health ecology with an understanding of system interactions. Such persons must develop the skills to design, implement, and administer health care prevention and environmental protection programs, a few of which are described below.

10. Residential complexes should be established for those aged who cannot maintain a residence, although every attempt should be made to allow the elderly to care for themselves. For those who require institutionalization, a range of facilities should be made available to fit the needs of individuals along a housing-health continuum. Medical care should be integrated into such complexes (or through home care if the aged prefer to live at home).

11. Public and private health care financing programs should permit payment to the healer of the patient's choice, in a setting of mutual choice by the healer and the patient, irrespective of the treatment modality of benefit sought and offered. Accordingly, such plans, whether public or private, should eliminate restrictive definitions of "provider," and of a "health benefit" and should further provide ready access without or with minimal deterrents such as "deductibles" and "co-insurance." (This is potentially a problem area because of the lack of cost controls. However, if there are fewer healers and hospital beds, demand can be controlled to some degree. Moreover, if health education works at all, demand should be far more closely calibrated with need then is now the case.)

12. An intensive effort must be made to further conceptualize our understanding of what health is, what new approaches should be tried, and what new concepts will underlie a new paradigm for the medicine of the future.

13. Investment in biomedical research oriented to techniques of prevention in *individual* cases should be expanded to ensure early detection of cancer, for example. A major focus of the program should be on detection and cure of degenerative diseases of old age, and alleviation, if not the cure, of chronic conditions.[2]

14. With the savings from decreased investments in the medical care system and in the training of physicians, and with such additional monies as are necessary (and will need to be provided initially), a substantial effort should be made to eliminate and mitigate the social and environmental causes of mortality and morbidity through the development of a wide range of *aggregate* prevention programs. A few examples would be:

- If funds spent on mass transit reduced the number of motor vehicles by one-half by 2000, perhaps as many as 100,000 lives might be saved and countless days of disability avoided (as well as ill health from inhalation of gasoline exhaust vapors).

- Accident prevention programs (including such simple expedients as imposing ceilings on the number of vehicles allowed on the road) would greatly reduce accidental trauma.

- If the projections of Lave and Seskin (and others) are reasonably accurate, reductions in air pollution alone would have a substantial impact on health status by the year 2000.

- Vastly expanded nutrition and food decontamination programs. We must first reorient biomedical research priorities to foster research on nutrition, and other factors such as noise, housing, biofeedback, and then, with the new information available, strengthen educational programs and heighten controls over food production and distribution.

- A "new towns" program to create smaller communities with presumably less stress and congestion may reduce levels or morbidity associated with either or both physical and mental conditions.

- Our approach to commerce and industry in terms of the physical and psychic demands made upon personnel should be transformed to create more congenial, less stress-inducing conditions. This will be more easily facilitated when people begin to understand how to achieve and maintain their health. The efforts of Saab and Volvo in Sweden to expand the responsibility of each worker are examples. Companies in the United States, including General Foods, Procter and Gamble, and Scott Paper Company, have also begun to do the same. More should follow suit, and much more experimentation must take place.

- Comprehensive fluoridation programs have demonstrated, at little cost, that the incidence of tooth decay and oral diseases can be reduced.
- Research and development programs in biomedical fields should be forced to focus on the causes of disease rather than on the elaboration of curative weaponry. An example was given earlier—a shift in biomedical research priorities to nutritional research at the expense of artificial knuckle joints.

15. Finally, we must have sweeping institutional change. At the most fundamental level, health will always be unequally distributed if other resources are unequally distributed. Poverty not only creates disease, it constricts and even strangles the opportunity to pursue health. Unquestionably, economic inequality is unhealthy. But even within the constraints of an existing economic order, there are measures that could be taken to redeploy our institutions to aid in the search for health. For example:

- The working day could be staggered so that traffic and other congestion could be minimized and persons given options to work at times more congenial to them.
- Schools, hospitals, and other public buildings, and even multiple dwellings could be redesigned to maximize healthful interactions and conditions. Examples include redesigning living spaces to promote interactions

among people through the use of common areas and facilities, the maximization of natural light, and the reduction or elimination of stress-producing noise.

- Through reconceptualization of land use priorities, the means could be found to create more open recreational spaces, including bike and hiking paths, tennis courts, and so on.

- The productive capacities of the aging, who will increase in numbers, could be used if the elderly were permitted to continue to work if they wished. One way to facilitate this would be to open up the job market so that younger workers could leave their jobs for one or two years and then return.

This is just a start; much more is required.

A SCENARIO FOR A NEW MEDICINE

In the year 2000 there will still be a medical care system, but it will be smaller than at present and will consume far fewer resources, relatively. The system will be organized around three types of facilities. The first is the neighborhood hospital and learning center, with fully staffed and equipped emergency care facilities. The hospital will have emergency facilities, a large outpatient department for ambulatory care, and a learning center for general use by providers and consumers alike. The learning center will offer classes and seminars in health and provide outreach services as well. Up-to-date health information will be available, as well as free consultations with trained personnel on health and treatment problems.

All neighborhood hospitals will be community owned and managed. Beyond the emergency facilities, no other specifications will be imposed. Further, admissions to the hospital will be made only on a voluntary basis and hospital privileges will not be limited to trained personnel.

The second key facility is the regional health center. Costly and sophisticated treatment will be provided here, only on an inpatient basis. Referrals will be made to the regional center from the neighborhood facilities.

Residential complexes for the elderly, incorporating care, will be the third type of facility. These facilities will stress self-care and responsibility but will provide all necessary medical care on site.

Health care personnel in 2000 will no longer be rigidly stratified by training levels. Rather, health care teams will replace the solo physician, followed by his or her faithful assistants. All teams will be hospital-based, although they will be deployed in emergency situations. There will be no independent office practice; all practitioners, however trained or with whatever skills, will practice in hospital or home settings. There will be no licensure restrictions, although a system of certification will require that all persons proposing to provide care furnish all pertinent information to patients, including training and experience, costs, treatment philosophy, and techniques to be used.

The personnel engaged in health will differ greatly in social, education, and demographic terms from those currently dominating the profession. Most will be trained in health or human ecology; few will be trained as physicians are now trained. Most training will be experiential, although the need for some didactic teaching will remain. No qualifications for training will be imposed, but the completion of training will not ensure placement with a hospital.

Astride the system will be the Department of Health Affairs. The mission of this department will be to maintain the environment in a manner as conducive to health as possible. Naturally, there will be conflicts between the Department and other agencies, institutions, and organizations desiring to engage in activities that pose dangers to the environment. But the department will possess the power to abate activities until a full assessment of the health impact of the activity can be made.

The department will work closely with agencies providing biomedical research support. Biomedical research will accordingly be refocused on social and environmental factors related to health. At the local level, citizens will control their own health care systems, featuring the neighborhood hospital and learning center. Each community will be given the necessary resources to design and implement health programs, subject only to broad specifications. Each citizen will have access to those drugs and tools of care necessary for treatment. Tools too costly to deploy at the local level or drugs for which citizens have not been given sufficient information will be available only at the regional health center. Health care will be federally underwritten but largely on a bloc grant basis. In addition to grants to neighborhoods and regions, grants will also be made available for experimental projects on either a local or regional basis. Participation by healers and patients will be voluntary.

This may not sound very different, but given where medicine is today and the trajectory it is on, to accomplish this much by the year 2000 will be remarkable, even if it is only the first step toward health.

Notes and References

CHAPTER 2

1. See E. A. Codman, "The Product of the Hospital," *Surgery, Gynecology and Obstetrics,* **18** (1914), 491–496.

2. Robert S. McCleery, et al., *One Life—One Physician* (New York: The Public Interest Press, 1971).

3. See C. E. Lewis, "Variations in Incidence of Surgery," *New England Journal of Medicine,* **281,** 6 (October 16, 1969), 880–884.

4. John P. Bunker, "Surgical Manpower," *New England Journal of Medicine,* **282,** 3 (January 15, 1970).

5. See Lincoln Moses and Frederick Mosteller, "Institutional Differences in Post-Operative Death Rates," *Journal of the American Medical Association,* **162,** 7 (October 13, 1956).

6. See Robert H. Brook, M.D., Sc.D., et al., "Effectiveness of Non-Emergency Care via an Emergency Room," *Annals of Internal Medicine,* **78** (1973).

7. Ninety to 95 percent of the medical resident staff at that time were affiliated with the highly regarded Johns Hopkins University School of Medicine, and were graduates of American medical schools.

8. See Brook, footnote 6, this chapter.

9. David Kessner, M.D., et al., unpublished report of the Institute of Medicine, National Academy of Sciences, n.d.

10. See, for example, John Williamson, M.D., "Evaluating Quality of Patient Care," *Journal of the American Medical Association,* **218,** 4 (October 25, 1971).

11. See, for example, R. E. Trussel, M. A. Morehead, et al., "A Study of the Quality of Hospital Care Secured by a Sample of Teamster Family Members in the New York Area." New York, School of Public Health and Administration Medicine, Columbia University, 1972. See also Barbara Starfield and David Scheff, "Effectiveness of Pediatric Care: The Relationship Between Process and Outcome," *Pediatrics,* **49,** 4 (April 1972).

12. See National Center for Health Statistics, *Statistics of the Bureau of Health and Vital Statistics,* Vol. 7, no. 2, February 1968.

13. *Christian Science Monitor,* **138,** 98.

14. See H. E. Evans, "Tonsillectomy and Adenoidectomy: Review of Published Evidence For and Against T. & A.," *Clinical Pediatrics,* **7,** 2 (February 1968), 71–75.

15. See footnote 12, this chapter.

16. See Pearay L. Ogra, M.D.: "Effect of Tonsillectomy and Adenoidectomy on Nasopharyngeal Antibody Response to Poliovirus," *New England Journal of Medicine,* **284,** (January 14, 1971), 59–64.

17. See, for example, Samuel D. Lipton, "On Psychology of Childhood Tonsillectomy," *Psychoanalytic Study of the Child,* **17** (1962), 363–417.

18. James C. Doyle, "Unnecessary Ovariectomies," *Journal of the American Medical Association,* **148,** 13 (1952); and "Unnecessary Hysterectomies: Study of 6,248 Operations in 35 hospitals in 1948," *Journal of the American Medical Association,* **151** (1963), 360–365.

19. In the case of chloramphenicol, routine oral use results in 1:10,000 deaths from anemia. Despite this fact the drug is still prescribed. See California State Department of Public Health, Senate Committee, "Fatal Aplastic Anemia in California, Its Relationship to the Drug Chloramphenicol," November 23, 1962.

20. *Minneapolis Tribune,* October 16, 1972.

21. Seymour Handler, M.D., "Bring Back the Mustard Plaster," *Minnesota Medicine,* **54** (December 1971), 973–979.

22. Charlotte Muller, "The Over-Medicated Society: Forces in the Marketplace for Medical Care," *Science,* **176** (May 5, 1972), 488.

23. For a comprehensive treatment, see R. H. Moser, *Diseases of Medical Progress: A Study of Iatrogenic Disease,* 3d ed. (Springfield, Ill.: Charles C Thomas, 1969).

24. John Pekkanen, *The American Connection* (Chicago: Follett Publishing Co., 1973).

25. *Ibid.,* pp. 84–85.

26. See U.S. Department of Health, Education, and Welfare, *Report of the Secretary's Commission on Medical Malpractice* (Washington, D.C.: U.S. Government Printing Office, 1973).

27. See R. W. Quinn and E. S. Campbell, "Heart Disease in Children: Survey of School Children in Nashville, Tennessee," *Yale Journal of Biology and Medicine,* **34** (1962), 370–385.

28. See A. B. Bergman and S. J. Stamm, "The Morbidity of Cardiac Non-Disease in Schoolchildren," *New England Journal of Medicine,* **276,** 18 (May 4, 1967), 1008.

29. For a good treatment of this point, see J. Ralph Audy, M.D., Ph.D., "Man-Made Maladies and Medicine," *California Medicine,* November 1970, 48.

30. Ivan Illich, *Medical Nemesis* (London: Calder and Boyars, 1974).

31. See A. K. Shapiro, "The Placebo Effect in the History of Medical Treatment: Implications for Psychiatry," *American Journal of Psychiatry,* **116** (1959), 293. For a general discussion of the placebo, see Frederick Evans, "The Power of a Sugar Pill," *Psychology Today,* April 1974.

32. Jerome Frank, *Persuasion and Healing* (New York: Schocken Books, 1961), p. 66.

33. *Ibid.,* p. 67.

34. F. A. Folgyesi, "School for Patients," *British Journal of Medical Hypnotism,* **5** (1954), 5.

35. See Frank, *Persuasion and Healing,* p. 70. See also H. R. Lewis and M. E. Lewis, *Psychosomatics* (New York: Viking Press, 1972), pp. 106–109.

36. For a comprehensive and critical assessment of the research on the "Hawthorne effect," see Henry A. Landsberger, *Hawthorne Revisited* (Ithaca, N.Y.: Cornell University Press, 1958).

37. Arthur Young, quoted in Handler, footnote 21 (this chapter), p. 973.

38. Lewis Thomas, M.D., "Guessing and Knowing," *Saturday Review,* **55,** 52 (January 1973). By permission of SR Publishing Assets, Inc. (Emphasis added.)

39. Cochrane for one does not agree. See A. L. Cochrane, CBE, FREP, *Effectiveness and Efficiency* (London: The Nuffield Provincial Hospitals Trust, 1972).

40. Allen Chase, *The Biological Imperative* (New York: Holt, Rinehart and Winston, 1972).

41. *The Los Angeles Times,* November 6, 1972.

42. Unpublished data, National Center for Health Statistics, based on 1971 data.

43. See footnote 39, this chapter.

44. One major study, for example, followed 176 cases of confirmed cancer that regressed without treatment. See T. D. Eversa and W. H. Cole, *Spontaneous Regression of Cancer* (Philadelphia: W. B. Saunders Co., 1966).

45. See, for example, Thomas McKeown, *Time Trend Studies* (London: Oxford University Press and Nuffield Press, 1971). The authors trace the rise and fall of disease conditions as they are influenced by social and environmental factors.

46. See footnote 73, Chapter 3.

47. René Dubos, *Man, Medicine & Environment* (New York: Praeger, 1968), p. 78. © by Encyclopaedia Britannica. Excerpted and reprinted by permission of Praeger Publishers, Inc.

48. John Powles, "On the Limitations of Modern Medicine," *Science, Medicine and Man,* **1** (1973), 1–30. Headington Hill Hall, Oxford, England: Pergamon Press, Ltd. Used by permission of Pergamon Press, Ltd.

49. John C. Cassel, M.D., "Health Consequences of Population and Crowding," paper presented at the AMA Congress of Environmental Health, Los Angeles, California, April 24–25, 1972.

50. See, for example, Richard Auster, Irving Leveson, and Deborah Sarachek, "The Production of Health; An Exploratory Study," *Journal of Human Resources*, **4,** 4 (Fall 1969); and Victor Fuchs, "The Contribution of Health Services to the American Economy," *Milbank Memorial Fund Quarterly*, **44,** 4 (October 1966).

51. The research, done by Auster, Leveson, and Sarachek (see footnote 50) is reported in Victor Fuchs, *The Service Economy* (New York: National Bureau of Economic Research, 1968).

52. The findings of the study are reported in *Drug Research Reports*, **15,** 47 (November 22, 1972), 6.

53. Charles T. Stewart, Jr., "Allocation of Resources to Health," *Journal of Human Resources*, **6,** 2, 105.

54. Eli Ginzberg, *Men, Money, and Medicine* (New York: Columbia University Press, 1969).

55. *Journal of the Mount Sinai Hospital of New York*, **19** (March/April 1953), 734.

56. Ginzberg, footnote 54 (this chapter), p. 23.

57. Victor Fuchs, "Some Economic Aspects of Mortality in Developed Countries," paper presented to the International Economic Association Conference on Economics of Health and Medical Care, Tokyo, April 2–7, 1973.

58. Carl E. Taylor, M.D., and Nevin Scrimshaw, *Interactions of Nutrition and Infection* (Geneva: World Health Organization, 1968).

59. What little work there is was reviewed by Robert N. Grosse in "Cost-Benefit Analysis of Health Services," *The Annals of the American Academy of Political and Social Science*, **399** (January 1972), 89.

60. *Ibid.*, p. 98.

61. See, for example, May Tuma and N. Tuma, "Schizophrenia—An Experimental Study of Five Treatment Methods," *British Journal of Psychiatry*, **111** (June 1965), 505–510.

62. U.S. Department of Health, Education, and Welfare, Public Health Service, *Mental Health* (Washington, D.C.: U.S. Government Printing Office, 1969), pp. 193–197.

63. *Ibid.*, p. 195.

CHAPTER 3

1. Oliver Wendell Holmes, Sr., *Medical Essays* (Boston: Houghton Mifflin, 1892), p. 202.

2. Lord Ritchie-Calder, *Medicine and Man* (New York: Signet Science Library, 1958), p. 47. By permission of the author.

3. *Ibid.*, p. 57.

4. Lawrence J. Henderson, quoted in Herrman L. Blumgart, "Caring for the Patient," *New England Journal of Medicine*, **270** (1964), 449.

5. The churches were first responsible for hospital construction, but more as a haven for the homeless than a place for the provision of care. My reference is to the "modern" hospital, focused on the provision of care to the sick. For a general history of hospitals, see Mary Risley, *House of Healing: The Story of the Hospital* (Garden City, N.Y.: Doubleday, 1961).

6. For a discussion of institution building, see David Rothman, *The Discovery of the Asylum* (Boston: Little, Brown, 1971).

7. Kerr White, "Health Care Arrangements in the United States: A.D. 1972," in "Medical Care and Medical Cure," *Milbank Memorial Fund Quarterly*, **50**, Part 2, no. 4 (October 1972), 19. By permission of the Milbank Memorial Fund.

8. René Dubos, *Mirage of Health* (New York: World Perspectives, Harper & Row, 1959).

9. See, for example, Floyd W. Matson, *The Broken Image* (Garden City, N.Y.: Doubleday Anchor Books, 1966), p. 14.

10. William Irwin Thompson, "Planetary Vistas," *Harpers*, **243** (December 1971), 73.

11. Michael G. Michaelson, "The Failure of American Medicine," *The American Scholar*, **39**, 4 (Autumn 1970), 702. Copyright © 1970 by the United Chapters of Phi Beta Kappa. By permission of the publishers.

12. Russell Roth, M.D., *The AMA News*, March 27, 1972.

13. René Dubos, *Man, Medicine, & Environment* (New York: Praeger, 1968). p. 66 (copyright by Encyclopaedia Britannica).

14. Based on medical specialty trends and current residents in training, the number of physicians who practice as specialists will increase from roughly 50 percent today to 55 percent in 1980. This increase caps a steady increase in both the number of specialty categories recognized by the AMA and number of specialists. See workpaper, "Medical Manpower Specialty Distribution Projections: 1975 and 1980," Health Services Research Center, Institute for Interdisciplinary Studies, May 1971.

15. See Eliot Freidson, *Profession of Medicine* (New York: Dodd, Mead, 1970), p. 251.

16. Kerr White, footnote 7 (this chapter), p. 37.

17. The term "fragmentation" in this context means at least two things: first, that medical care is provided by many individuals, groups, and institutions. And second, health manpower is classified by rigid licensure laws resulting in the lack of a rational pattern of manpower deployment and utilization.

18. American Medical Association, "Distribution of Physicians in the U.S., 1970," Center for Health Services Research and Development,

Chicago, 1971. See also Committee for Economic Development, "Building a National Health-Care System," New York, April 1973.

19. See National Health Survey data, especially since 1968 when the Medicaid legislation was implemented.

20. *Santa Barbara News Press,* December 2, 1972.

21. See footnote 14, this chapter.

22. Eliot Freidson, *Professional Dominance* (New York: Atherton Press, 1971).

23. Eliot Freidson, "Professionalism: The Doctor's Dilemma," *Social Policy,* January/February 1971, 37.

24. See, for example, H. G. Mather et al., "Acute Myocardial Infarction: Home and Hospital Treatment," *British Medical Journal,* **3** (1971), 334–338.

25. Irving K. Zola, "Medicine as an Institution of Social Control." A paper presented at the Medical Sociology Conference of the British Sociological Conference, Westen-Super Mare, November 5–7, 1971.

26. David Mechanic, "Health and Illness in Technological Societies," *Hastings Center Studies,* **1**, 3 (1973), 11.

27. See, for example, Kerr White, M.D., et al., "International Comparisons of Medical Care Utilization," *New England Journal of Medicine,* **272** (1967), 516–522.

28. *Time,* January 10, 1967, p. 42.

29. See, for example, Kerr White, M.D., "Medical Care Research on Health Care Systems," *Journal of Medical Education,* **42** (August 1967), 729; and Milton I. Roemer, M.D., *Medical Care in Relation to Public Health, A Monograph* (Geneva: World Health Organization, 1957).

30. In Great Britain, more than 97 percent of the population receives its care from the National Health Service.

31. A thorough comparative review of the health care systems in the United States, England, and Sweden can be found in Odin W. Anderson, *Health Care: Can There Be Equity?* (New York: Wiley-Interscience, 1973).

32. See U.S. Department of Commerce, Bureau of the Census, *Statistical Abstract of the United States,* 94th ed. (Washington, D.C.: U.S. Government Printing Office, 1973).

33. Although the percentage of GNP spent for medical care may be relatively the same among countries, the "real" dollars expended for health care may vary greatly because of what various currencies will buy.

34. The phenomenon of the multinational corporation has been widely reported in recent years. See, for example, *Newsweek,* November 20, 1972, and Peter Drucker, "The New Markets and the New Capitalism," *The Public Interest,* Fall 1970, 44.

35. The World Health Organization (WHO) has assumed the responsibility for international disease control, but is so hemmed in by world politics and the constraints in its mandate that its impact is limited.

36. These data are drawn from Colin Fraser Brockington, *World Health* (Baltimore: Penguin Books, 1958), p. 30.

37. *Ibid.*, p. 29.

38. Gunnar Myrdal, *Asian Drama: An Inquiry into the Poverty of Nations.* Abridged. A Condensation by Seth S. King of the Twentieth Century Fund Study. © 1971 by The Twentieth Century Fund, New York. Published by Vintage Books, A Division of Random House, New York.

39. *Ibid.*, pp. 375–376. Used by permission of Twentieth Century Fund.

40. John Bryant, *Health and the Developing World* (Ithaca, N.Y.: Cornell University Press, 1969), p. 35.

41. *Ibid.*, p. 35.

42. See *ibid.*, p. 44.

43. Brian Abel-Smith, *An International Study of Health Expenditure* (Geneva: World Health Organization, 1967).

44. *Santa Barbara News and Review*, January 27, 1973.

45. The research is reported in Thelma Moss and Kendall Johnson, "The Body Is an Energy Field," *Harpers*, January 1973.

46. See, for example, Rolf Alexander, *Creative Realism* (New York: Pageant Press, 1954); and Elmer E. Green, Ph.D., "How to Make Use of the Field of Mind Theory," in *The Dimensions of Healing: A Symposium*, The American Academy of Parapsychology and Medicine, 1973, p. 41.

47. Perhaps the best source of information on auras and Kirlian photography is S. Krippner and D. Rubin (eds.), *Galaxies of Life: The Human Aura in Acupuncture and Kirlian Photography* (New York: Gordon and Breach, 1973).

48. See, for example, Shafica Karagula, M.D., *Breakthrough to Creativity* (Los Angeles: DeVorss and Co., Inc., 1967).

49. Andrew Weil, *The Natural Mind* (Boston: Houghton Mifflin, 1972), p. 173.

50. Rick J. Carlson, *The Frontiers of Science & Medicine*, proceedings of a conference. London, May, 1974. (Wildwood House, London, 1975).

51. See Ronald Melzack, Ph.D., "How Acupuncture Works: A Sophisticated Western Theory Takes the Mystery Out," *Psychology Today*, June 1973, 28. See also John W. White, "Acupuncture: The World's Oldest System of Medicine," *Psychic*, July 1972; and *The Dimensions of Healing: A Symposium* (San Francisco: The American Academy of Parapsychology and Medicine, 1973), pp. 159, 168.

52. *The Varieties of Healing Experiences*, transcript of the Interdisciplinary Symposium of The American Academy of Parapsychology and Medicine, San Francisco, October 30, 1971.

53. See footnote 51, this chapter.

54. See Elmer E. Green, "Biofeedback for Mind-Body Self-Regulation: Healing and Creativity," *The Varieties of Healing Experiences,* footnote 51, p. 29. See also a new book on Arigo by John G. Fuller, *Arigo: Surgeon of the Rusty Knife* (New York: Thomas Y. Crowell, 1974).

55. See Green, footnote 46 and footnote 54 (this chapter), pp. 45–47.

56. See, for example, Theodore Barber et al. (eds.), *Biofeedback and Self-Control* (Chicago: Aldine Publishing Company, 1971); and Leo V. DiCara, "Learning in the Autonomic Nervous System," *Scientific American,* January 1970, 30–39. See also Barbara Brown, *New Mind, New Body* (New York: Harper & Row, 1974).

57. Robert Ornstein, *The Psychology of Consciousness* (New York: Viking Press, 1972). p. 200.

58. See Thomas H. Budzynski, Johann Stoyva, and Charles Adler, "Feedback-Induced Muscle Relaxation: Application to Tension Headaches," *Journal of Behavioral Therapy and Experimental Psychology,* 1 (1970), 205–211. See also Leo V. DiCara, "Learning in the Autonomic Nervous System," *Scientific American,* January 1970, 30–39.

59. This information was drawn from "A Study of Psychic Surgery and Spiritual Healing in the Philippines," an unpublished report, July 1973. See also Harold Sherman, *Wonder Healers of the Philippines* (London: Psychic Press, 1967), and Thomas Valentine, *Psychic Surgery* (Chicago: Henry Regnery Company, 1973).

60. Jerome Frank, *Persuasion and Healing* (New York: Schocken Books, 1961).

61. See, for example, K. N. Udupa and R. H. Singh, "The Scientific Basis of Yoga," *Journal of the American Medical Association,* **222,** 10 (June 5, 1972).

62. Steven Brena, M.D., *Yoga and Medicine* (New York: Julian Press, Inc., 1972).

63. For a discussion of some of these studies, see Ornstein, footnote 57 (this chapter). See also Robert K. Wallace and Herbert Benson, "The Physiology of Meditation," *Scientific American,* **226** (February 1972), and the April 1974 issue of *Psychology Today,* which contains three articles on meditation in which many studies of physiological impacts of meditation are reviewed.

64. See footnotes 50 and 52 (this chapter) for a discussion of Simonton's work.

65. Allopathic medicine is dominant in the United States, but there are residual practices based on differing theories. Chiropractic, for example, stresses the importance of maintaining equilibrium in the body and relies heavily on bodily manipulation to achieve its results. The practice of osteopathy is somewhat similar to chiropractic, but has been mostly absorbed into the mainstream of modern allopathic medicine.

Homeopathy, in sharper contrast to allopathy, relies on medicinals that are the same as, or similar to, the "agents" of the disease for which a cure is sought. For a description of homeopathy, see George Vithoulkas, *Homeopathy: Medicine of the New Man* (New York: Avon, 1971).

66. This dichotomy between traditional Chinese medicine and modern medical practice is comprehensibly described in *Away With All Pests* by Dr. Joshua S. Horn (New York: Modern Reader Paperback, 1971). See also M. H. Liang et al., "Chinese Health Care: Determinants of the System," *American Journal of Public Health*, **63**, 2 (February 1973), 102. And see Paul T. K. Lin, "Medicine in China," *The Center Magazine*, May/June 1974.

67. See, for example, F. M. Alexander, *The Use of Self* (Manchester: Re-educational Publications, Ltd., 1932).

68. See, for example, G. E. Caghill, "Appreciation: The Educational Methods of F. M. Alexander," in F. M. Alexander, *The Unusual Constant in Living* (New York: Dutton, 1941); and R. A. Dart, "An Anatomist's Tribute to F. M. Alexander," *South Africa Medical Journal*, **21** (1947), 74.

69. *Science*, **185** (July 5, 1974), 20–27.

70. *The Budget of the U.S. Government, Fiscal Year 1975* (Washington, D.C.: U.S. Government Printing Office, 1974), p. 197.

71. Stephen P. Strickland, *Politics, Science, and Dread Disease* (Cambridge: Commonwealth Fund Book, Harvard University Press, 1972), p. 1. © 1972 by Harvard University. By permission of the Harvard University Press.

72. *Ibid.,* p. 272.

73. The "limitation" of tuberculosis is somewhat open to question. A number of observers have pointed out that the ravages of TB were on the wane—largely through changes in the socioenvironment—long before the advent of TB "treatment." See, for example, René Dubos, *White Plague: Tuberculosis, Man and Society* (Boston: Little, Brown, 1952).

74. See footnote 71, this chapter.

75. Philip Nobile, "King Cancer," *Esquire*, June 1973.

76. *Ibid.,* p. 105.

77. *Ibid.*

78. See Brockington, *World Health*, footnote 36, this chapter. See also Nobile, "King Cancer," footnote 75, this chapter; and Henry Lynch, M.D. (ed.), *Cancer and You* (Springfield, Ill.: Charles C Thomas, 1971), particularly Chapter 4, where the author enumerates many known and suspected causes of cancer.

79. Some of the origins and variations in cancer peculiar to geography and culture are traced in Vilhjalmur Stefansson, *Cancer: Disease of Civiliza-*

tion (New York: Hill & Wang, 1960). See also the preceding section on the international context for medical care.

80. See U.S. Department of Health, Education, and Welfare, National Institute of Health, National Cancer Institute, *The National Cancer Program Plan* (Washington, D.C.: U.S. Government Printing Office, 1973).

81. See interview with Dr. Frank J. Rauscher, National Cancer Institute, *U.S. News and World Report,* December 4, 1972, 38.

82. Nobile, "King Cancer," footnote 75 (this chapter), p. 210.

83. *Ibid.,* p. 210.

CHAPTER 4

1. Herman Kahn, *The Year 2000: A Framework for Speculation on the Next Thirty-Three Years* (New York: Macmillan, 1967).

2. Charles Hampden-Turner, *Radical Man* (Cambridge: Schenkman Publishing Co., 1970), pp. 305–306 (emphasis in the original). © 1971 Schenkman Publishing Co., Inc., Cambridge, Mass. 02138. Reprinted with permission.

3. U.S. Department of Commerce, Bureau of the Census, *Statistical Abstract of the United States,* 94th ed. (Washington, D.C.: U.S. Government Printing Office, 1973), p. 48.

4. *Ibid.,* p. 42.

5. The Commission on Population Growth and the American Future reported its results to President Nixon, who summarily disagreed with them. The Report strongly argues for a policy of population stabilization. The Commission has continued to publicize its findings, although on a "private" basis.

6. Unfortunately, demographic predictions are often infirm bases for action; they often prove to be inaccurate. George Grier of the Washington Center for Metropolitan Studies argues that "The 1970 census counts revealed a change . . . exactly the opposite of what was expected." (*Minneapolis Tribune,* June 25, 1973). See his *The Changing Age Profile, Implications for Policy Planning in Metropolitan Washington* (Washington, D.C.: Washington Center for Metropolitan Studies, 1964).

7. The quotation is attributed to Dr. Comfort by Gordon Rattray Taylor in *The Biological Time Bomb* (New York: World Publishing Company, 1968), p. 92.

8. Alexander Comfort, *The Process of Aging* (London: Weidenfelt & Nicholson, 1964).

9. There is some research supporting the point. Recent NIH studies reveal that the "aging" break where psychological functions begin to deteriorate is shifting from the early to the late 60s.

10. Telephone conversation with AMA representative, May 11, 1972.

11. The population under 19, 77,150,000, was derived from U.S. Department of Commerce, Bureau of the Census, "Projections of the Population of the United States, by Age and Sex: 1970 to 2020," *Current Population Reports,* Series P-25, no. 470 (Washington, D.C.: U.S. Government Printing Office, 1971), p. 55.

12. See, for example, Ethel Shanas, *The Health of Older People* (Cambridge: Harvard University Press, 1962) and "Health of Older People," Statistical Bulletin, New York, Metropolitan Life Insurance Company, September 1971. For a general discussion of the health problems of the aging, see Edward J. Stieglitz, *The Second Forty Years* (Philadelphia: J. B. Lippincott Co., 1946).

13. See U.S. Department of Health, Education, and Welfare, Social Security Administration, Office of Research and Statistics, *Compendium of National Health Expenditures Data* (Washington, D.C.: U.S. Government Printing Office, 1972).

14. Naturally this calculation has defects. For example, the 9.2 percent per year increase may not hold because backlogged health care needs by the aged may be decreasing now that Medicare has been in effect for eight years. Moreover, the 2 trillion figure is relative to other expenditures and is the product of a simple linear projection. The cutting question, which is very difficult to calculate, is what percentage of GNP will be consumed by medical care expenditures, and of that how much will be allocated to the care of the elderly. It will probably be large, but it is impossible to predict the exact levels.

15. See U.S. Department of Health, Education, and Welfare, Public Health Service, *Health Resources Statistics, 1972–73* (Washington, D.C.: U.S. Government Printing Office, 1973).

16. Alvin Toffler, *Future Shock* (New York: Random House, 1970).

17. Donald Schoen, *Beyond the Stable State* (New York: Random House, 1971).

18. See, for example, Hans Selye, *The Stress of Life* (New York: McGraw-Hill, 1956).

19. From *Man, Medicine and Environment,* by René Dubos, p. 80. © 1968 by Encyclopaedia Brittanica. Excerpted and reprinted by permission of Praeger Publishers, Inc., New York.

20. *Ibid.,* p. 88.

21. John C. Cassel and Alexander H. Leighton, "Epidemiology and Mental Health" in *Mental Health Considerations in Public Health,* Public Health Service Publication 1898 (Washington, D.C., Government Printing Office, May, 1969), p. 67.

22. Kasl, Cobb, and Brooks traced increases in serum uric acid and cholesterol levels associated with loss of employment. See Stanley V. Kasl, Ph.D., Sidney Cobb, M.D., and George W. Brooks, M.P.H.,

"Changes in Serum Uric Acid and Cholesterol Levels in Men Undergoing Job Loss," *Journal of the American Medical Association,* **206,** 7 (November 11, 1968).

23. See footnote 21 (this chapter), p. 75.

24. These data are reported by Dodi Schultz, "The High Blood Pressure Time Bomb," *Viva,* April 1974.

25. Richard Rahe, Joseph McKean, Jr., and Ransom Arthur, "A Longitudinal Study of Life-Change and Illness Patterns," *Journal of Psychosomatic Research,* **10,** 4 (1967), 355. See also Ray H. Rosenham et al., "A Predictive Study of Coronary Heart Disease," *Journal of the American Medical Association,* **189** (1964), 15.

26. J. H. Holmes and M. Masuda, "Psychosomatic Syndrome," *Psychology Today,* April 1972, 71. See also research by G. W. Brown and J. L. Birley, "Crises and Life Changes and the Onset of Schizophrenia," *Journal of Health and Social Behavior,* **9** (September 1968), 203–214.

27. See Stanley V. Kasl and Sidney Cobb, "Effects of Parental Status Incongruence and Discrepancy on Physical and Mental Health of Adult Offspring," *Journal of Personality and Social Psychology,* **7,** 2 (October 1967).

28. James K. Skipper, Jr., and Robert C. Leonard, "Children, Stress and Hospitalizations: A Field Experiment," *Journal of Health and Social Behavior,* **9** (1968), 278.

29. See footnote 80, Chapter 3.

30. See Demetri B. Shimkin, "Man, Ecology and Health," *Archives of Environmental Health,* **20** (January 1970); and A. J. Klebba, "Mortality Trends in the U.S. 1954–1963," publ. 1000, ser. 20, no. 2 (Washington, D.C.: Public Health Service, 1965).

31. A paper presented by Gerald L. Looney, "Getting What We Pay For," at the Third Annual Meeting of the Comprehensive Health Planning Council of Maricopa County, Phoenix, Arizona, November 19, 1971.

32. Unfortunately, escaping the carnage through cycling instead of driving is unpromising; in 1965 more than 700 persons died in accidents while cycling. See "Reports of the Division of Vital Statistics," National Center for Health Statistics, 1967.

33. See U.S. National Health Survey, 1963, Series B, no. 37, pp. 20, 26.

34. Chase, footnote 39, Chapter 2.

35. U.S. Department of Health, Education, and Welfare, *National Institute of Alcohol Abuse and Alcoholism Report* (Washington, D.C.: U.S. Government Printing Office, February 1972.

36. These figures are understated—they include only reported addiction, a number far less than the number of addicted users. See *Statistical Abstract of the United States, 1973,* p. 83.

37. See "An Upturn in Smoking Despite All Warnings," *U.S. News and*

World Report, October 9, 1972, 92; and National Clearinghouse for Smoking and Health, Director of On-Going Research in Smoking and Health, *Report* (Washington, D.C.: Department of Health, Education, and Welfare, and Public Health Service, 1970), p. 229.

38. Based on DHEW projections, the United States will be graduating 12,000 physicians per year by 1975 as opposed to earlier annual crops of 8000.

39. This calculation is based on a gain of 1.48 gallons per capita to 2.37 gallons per capita from the period of 1940 to 1968.

40. See Arthur Freese, "Trauma: The Neglected Epidemic," *Saturday Review,* May 13, 1972, 58–62.

41. *Ibid.*

42. Chicago Hospital Council, "The Crisis in Emergency Care, Part 1. The Ambulance Scandal: A Hazard to Life and Health," *Medical World News,* **11** (December 4, 1970), 24.

43. Charles Frey, M.D., directed this research conducted at the University of Michigan. See Freese, footnote 40, this chapter.

44. *The Los Angeles Times,* November 20, 1972.

45. *Ibid.*

46. See Andrew Weil, *The Natural Mind* (Boston: Houghton Mifflin, 1973).

47. See interview with Jerome Jaffe, *Psychology Today,* August 1973.

48. Edward M. Brecher and the Editors of *Consumer Reports, Licit and Illicit Drugs* (Mount Vernon, N.Y.: Consumers Union, 1972).

49. Peter Koenig, "The Placebo Effect in Patent Medicine," *Psychology Today,* April 1973, 60.

50. Meadows, H., et al., *The Limits to Growth: A Report for the Club of Rome's Project on the Predicament of Mankind* (Washington, D.C.: Potomac Associates, 1972). Much of the Club's methodology is based on the work of Jay Forrester, principally his book *World Dynamics* (Cambridge: Wright-Allen Press, 1971).

51. Meadows et al., *The Limits to Growth,* p. 23.

52. Many observers feel that the Club of Rome has overstated its case. Among them is John Maddox, the editor of *Nature* magazine. See Maddox, *The Doomsday Syndrome* (New York: McGraw-Hill, 1972).

53. Barry Commoner, *The Closing Circle* (New York: Knopf, 1971). © 1971 by Barry Commoner. By permission of Alfred A. Knopf, Inc.

54. *Ibid.,* p. 189.

55. Garrett Hardin, "The Tragedy of the Commons," *Science,* **162** (December 13, 1968), 1243–1248. See also footnote 52, this chapter.

56. See, for example, Samuel S. Epstein, "Pollution and Health," in Michael P. Hamilton (ed.), *The New Genetics of the Future of Man* (Grand Rapids, Mich.: Eerdmans Publishing Company, 1972).

57. *Ibid.*, p. 183. By permission of Wm. B. Eerdmans Publishing Company.

58. See, for example, J. F. Cros, "Chemical Risk to Future Generations, *Scientist and Citizen*, **10** (1968), 113–117, and Report of the Advisory Panel on Mutagenicity, Report of the Secretary's Commission on Pesticides and Their Relationship to Environmental Health, DHEW, December 1969.

59. J. Lederberg, Foreword to Samuel S. Epstein and Marvin S. Legator (eds.), *The Mutagenicity of Pesticides: Concepts and Evaluation* (Cambridge: The MIT Press, 1971), p. x. By permission of The MIT Press.

60. See, for example, Theodore D. Sterling, "Air Pollution and Smoking," *Environment,* July/August 1973, 3.

61. E. C. Hammond and D. Horn, "Smoking and Death Rates: Report on Forty-four Months of Follow-Up of 186,763 Men," *Journal of the American Medical Association,* **166** (1958), 1294–1308.

62. P. Stocks, "On the Relations Between Atmospheric Pollution in Urban and Rural Localities and Mortality from Cancer, Bronchitis, and Pneumonia, with Particular Reference to 3, 4-Benayprene, Beryl-liu, Molybdenum, Vanadium, and Arsenic," *British Journal of Cancer,* **14** (1960), 397–418.

63. U.S. Surgeon General, *Report on Smoking and Health* (Washington, D.C.: U.S. Government Printing Office, 1964).

64. René Laennec pointed out the relationship between fossil-fuel use in industrial production and the contaminants that caused emphysema in 1819. Today fossil-fuel residues contribute only about 15 percent of the air pollution.

65. U.S. Surgeon General, *The Health Consequences of Smoking, A Public Health Service Review, 1967* (Washington, D.C.: Department of Health, Education, and Welfare, and Public Health Service, 1967), p. 26.

66. The Seventh Annual Public Health Service Report to the Congress on the Consequences of Cigarette Smoking, reported in the *New York Times,* January 18, 1973.

67. Sterling, footnote 60 (this chapter), p. 3.

68. Rachel Carson, *Silent Spring* (Boston: Houghton Mifflin, 1962).

69. M. Miettinen et al., "Effect of Cholesterol-Lowering Diet on Mortality from Coronary Heart Disease and Other Causes," *Lancet,* **2** (October 21, 1972), 835–838.

70. See J. B. Calhoun, "Population Density and Social Pathology," *Scientific American,* **206** (1962), 136. See also H. B. Andervont, "Influences of Environment on Mammary Cancer in Mice," *The Journal of the National Cancer Institute,* **4** (1964), 579–581. For more mixed results, see also a survey of research on crowding, *Psychology Today,* April 1974.

71. See Joseph R. Anticaglia and Alexander Cohen, "Extra-Auditory Effects of Noise as a Health Hazard," *American Industrial Hygiene Association,* **31** (1970), 277.

72. I. Abey-Wickrama, et al., "Mental Hospital Admissions and Noise," *The Lancet,* December 13, 1969, 1275.

73. Robert Baron, *The Tyranny of Noise* (New York: St. Martin's Press, 1970), p. 85. By permission of St. Martin's Press, Inc.

74. *Ibid.,* p. 56.

75. Commoner, footnote 53 (this chapter), p. 57.

76. See J. Ross McDonald, "Radiation in Aircraft," *Environment,* **15** (July/August 1973).

77. Susan Hopper (trans.), "Last Year at Deauville," *Environment,* **13** (July/August 1971), 36.

78. See "Don't Drink the Water," *Newsweek,* July 23, 1973, 48.

79. See, for example, Neville Grant, M.D., "Mercury in Man," *Environment,* **13** (May 1971), 3.

80. See, for example, Harvey Schroeder, "Metals in the Air," *Environment,* **13,** 8 (October 1971), 18.

81. The *Los Angeles Times,* September 28, 1972.

82. See, for example, a report of the U.S. Department of Labor, *Work in America* (Washington, D.C.: U.S. Government Printing Office, 1972).

83. Committee on Environmental Hazards of the American Academy of Pediatricians, "Acute and Chronic Childhood Lead Poisoning," *Pediatrics,* **47,** 5 (May 1971).

84. See *Science,* **181** (August 19, 1973), 534.

85. L. B. Lave and E. P. Seskin, "Air Pollution and Human Health," *Science,* **169,** 3947 (August 21, 1970).

86. Ronald Ridken, *Economic Costs of Air Pollution* (New York: Praeger, 1967). See also Committee of Public Health, "Air Pollution and Health," *The New York Academy of Medicine Bulletin,* **42,** 7 (July 1966).

87. René Dubos, "Promises and Hazards of Man's Adaptability," in Henry Jarrett (ed.), *Environmental Quality in a Growing Economy* (Baltimore: The Johns Hopkins University Press, 1966), p. 26 (emphasis added). Used by permission of Johns Hopkins Press.

88. Leo Srole, with Thomas S. Langner, Stanley T. Michael, Marvin K. Opler, and Thomas A. C. Rennie, *Mental Health in the Metropolis: Midtown Manhattan Study* (New York: McGraw-Hill, 1962). The study did *not* investigate matched institutional and noninstitutional populations. The inference, rather, rests on a comparison of the number of persons under treatment for diagnosed mental illness and the noninstitutionalized population studied.

89. Some of the major research includes: Benjamin Pasamanick (ed.), *Epidemiology of Mental Disorder* (Washington, D.C.: American Association for the Advancement of Science, 1959); A. B. Hollingshead and

F. C. Redlich, *Social Class and Mental Illness* (New York: John Wiley & Sons, Inc., 1958); P. Lemkau, C. Tietze, and M. Cooper, *Mental Hygiene in Public Health* (New York: McGraw-Hill, 1949); Thomas A. C. Rennie, Leo Srole, Marvin K. Opler, and Thomas S. Langner, "Urban Life and Mental Health," *American Journal of Psychiatry,* **113** (1957), 831; Leo Srole, Thomas S. Langner, and Thomas A. C. Rennie, "Mental Disorders in a Metropolis," *Public Health Report,* **72** (1957), 580; and E. W. Folile and J. E. Marches, "Mental Health Morbidity in a Suburban Community," *Journal of Clinical Psychology,* **24,** 1 (1968).

90. Brian Cooper, John Fry, and Graham Kalton, "A Longitudinal Study of Psychiatric Morbidity in a General Practice Population," *British Journal of Preventive and Social Medicine,* **23** (1969), 210.

91. On examination it is obvious that the studies used very different methodologies. As noted in L. Taylor and S. Chase, *Mental Health and Environment* (Harlow, Essex: Longmans, Green & Co., 1974), the disparities in results follow from examination of different phenomena: "The tables indicate then that the reported prevalence of mental disorder is largely a function of the intensity of the methods employed. In other words, the size of the catch depends upon the size of the mesh of the net that is used; mental institutions find the least, community services find more, and direct interviews find the most. Indeed, the over-enthusiastic psychiatric diagnostician can find evidence of psychiatric ill-health in most human beings; such findings perhaps tell us more about the observer than about those observed" (p. 177).

92. See, for example, Holmes and Masuda, footnote 26, this chapter.

93. Some of the works to which I have reference are *Imperial Animal* by Tiger and Robin Fox (New York: Holt, Rinehart and Winston, 1971); *The Naked Ape* by Morris (New York: McGraw-Hill, 1967); *African Genesis* by Ardry (New York: Atheneum, 1967); and *On Aggression* by Lorenz (New York: Harcourt Brace Jovanovich, 1966).

94. Konrad Lorenz, *Civilized Man's Eight Deadly Sins* (New York: Harcourt Brace Jovanovich, 1974).

95. Arthur Koestler, *The Ghost in the Machine* (New York: Macmillan, 1968).

96. See Srole, footnote 88 (this chapter), p. 362 (emphasis in original). Copyright by Leo Srole. By permission of Leo Srole and McGraw-Hill, Inc.

97. *Ibid.,* p. 362. Copyright by Leo Srole. By permission of Leo Srole and McGraw-Hill, Inc.

98. Herbert Goldhammer and Andrew Marshall, *Psychosis and Civilization* (Glencoe, Ill.: The Free Press, 1949).

99. *Ibid.,* p. 91.

100. Bruce P. Dohrenwend and Barbara S. Dohrenwend, *Social Status and Psychological Disorder: A Causal Inquiry* (New York: Wiley-Interscience, 1969).

101. Skinner's thesis is most cogently presented in *Beyond Freedom and Dignity* (New York: Knopf, 1971).

102. The use of psychoactive drugs is examined in Gerald L. Klerman, "Psychotropic Drugs as Therapeutic Agents," *Hastings Center Studies,* **2**, 1 (January 1974).

103. Robert Coles, "The Case of Michael Wechsler," *New York Review of Books,* May 18, 1972.

104. Ginzberg, footnote 53 (Chapter 2), pp. 229–230. By permission of the publisher.

105. Kai T. Erikson, *Wayward Pilgrims* (New York: John Wiley & Sons, 1966).

106. See, for example, Thomas Szasz, *The Manufacture of Madness* (New York: Harper & Row, 1970), and R. D. Laing, *The Politics of Experience* (New York: Ballantine, 1970). See also Edgar Z. Friedenburg, *Laing* (New York: Viking Press, 1974).

107. D. L. Rosenhans, "On Being Sane in Insane Places," *Science,* **19** (January 19, 1973).

108. The study is reported in *Society,* **9**, 10 (September/October 1972), and was done by E. Fuller Torrey. See also Frank, footnote 60, Chapter 3.

109. Oscar Newman, *Architectural Design for Crime Prevention* (Washington, D.C.: National Institute of Law Enforcement and Criminal Justice, 1973).

110. *The Los Angeles Times,* January 7, 1973.

111. Matthew Dumont, M.D., *The Absurd Healer* (New York: Viking Press, 1971).

112. *Ibid.,* p. 26. Dumont offers as support the Srole work, already cited, and M. Greenblatt, P. Emery, and B. Glueck, *Poverty and Mental Health,* Psychiatric Research Report no. 22 (Washington, D.C.: American Psychiatric Association, 1967), and Frank Riessman, Jerome Cohen, and Arthur Pearl (eds.), *Mental Health of the Poor: New Treatment Approaches for Low Income People* (New York: The Free Press, 1964).

113. Herman Kahn and Anthony J. Weiner, "The Next Thirty-Three Years: A Framework for Speculation," in Daniel Bell (ed.), *Toward the Year 2000: Work in Progress* (Boston: Daedalus Library, Beacon Press, 1967–1968), pp. 79–84.

114. Taylor, footnote 7 (this chapter), pp. 204–205.

115. Raul de Brigard and Olaf Helmer, "Some Potential Societal Developments 1970–2000," Report of Research, The Institute for the Future, IFF Report R-7, 1970.

116. *Budget of the United States Government* (Washington, D.C.: U.S. Government Printing Office, 1972), pp. 388, 391, 412. Of course, there are other biomedical expenditures. Allocations to NIH and NIMH constitute a little more than one-half of total federal support.

117. Much of the material in this section has been culled from a paper prepared by Robert Sinsheimer, Ph.D., a nuclear biologist at the California Institute of Technology, for a conference held at the Center for the Study of Democratic Institutions in May 1972.

118. *Ibid.*

119. For a discussion of amniocentisis see Amitai Etzioni, *Genetic Fix: New Opportunities and Dangers for You, Your Child and the Nation* (New York: Macmillan, 1973).

120. Some Australian researchers have reported a nearly successful implantation. And successful implantations have been reported in Great Britain. See *The New York Times,* July 16, 1974, p. 18, and September 15, 1974, sec. 6, p. 17.

121. *The New York Times,* January 11, 1973.

122. It is not clear whether the study controlled for other quality variables in the sample hospitals.

123. See Mather et al., footnote 24, chapter 3.

124. Anne Somers, "Health Care and the Political System," paper presented to the National Center for Health Service Research and Development Conference on Technology and Health Care Systems in the 1900s, Rockville, Maryland, January 19, 1972.

125. See Grosse, footnote 59, Chapter 2.

126. Freese, footnote 40, this chapter.

127. See footnote 31, this chapter.

128. See footnote 121, this chapter.

129. This section is derived from a monograph, "The Pursuit of Well-Being," co-authored Harvey Wheeler and R. J. Carlson, prepared for the Center for the Study of Democratic Institutions, February 1973. Most of the concepts are Dr. Wheeler's and credit is owed him.

130. See Abraham Maslow, *Toward a Psychology of Being* (New York: Van Nostrand, 1962); and Frank Goble, *The Third Force* (New York: Grossman Publishers, 1970).

131. See footnote 13, this chapter.

132. See footnote 82, this chapter.

133. *Ibid.*

134. J. B. Gordon, A. Ahman, and M. C. Brodis, *Industrial Safety Statistics: A Re-Examination* (New York: Praeger, 1971).

135. See, for example, Barry Commoner, "Workplace Burden," *Environment,* July/August 1973.

136. Demitri B. Shimkin, "Man, Ecology and Health," *Archives of Environmental Health,* **20** (January 1970), 115. Copyright 1970, American Medical Association. Used by permission of the American Medical Association.

137. See, for example, Myron J. Lefcowitz, "Poverty and Health: A Reexamination," *Inquiry,* **10** (March 1973).

138. P. B. Horton and G. K. Leslie, *The Sociology of Social Problems* (New York: Appleton-Century-Crofts, 1965), p. 585.

139. The data are drawn from Rodger L. Hurley, *Poverty and Mental Retardation* (New York: Random House, 1969).

CHAPTER 5

1. George Leonard, *The Transformation: A Guide to the Inevitable Changes in Humankind* (New York: Delacorte Press, 1972).

2. Thomas Kuhn, *The Structure of Scientific Revolutions* (Chicago: University of Chicago Press, 1962).

3. Leonard, footnote 133 (Chapter 4), p. 122.

4. Jonas Salk, *The Survival of the Wisest* (New York: Harper & Row, 1973).

5. *Ibid.,* p. 82. By permission of Harper & Row.

6. Ronald Segal, *The Struggle Against History* (New York: Bantam Books, 1973), p. 19.

7. Robert Theobald, *Habit and Habitat* (Englewood Cliffs, N.J.: Prentice-Hall, 1972), p. 1. © 1972 by Robert Theobald. By permission of Prentice-Hall, Inc.

8. N. Freedland, *The Occult Explosion* (London: Michael Joseph, 1972).

9. Colin Wilson, *The Occult* (New York: Vintage Books, 1973).

10. J. R. R. Tolkien, *The Lord of the Rings* (Boston: Houghton-Mifflin, 1965).

11. See, for example, Carlos Castaneda, *A Separate Reality* (New York: Simon & Schuster, 1971).

12. Jean Paul Sartre, *The Roads to Freedom* (New York: Knopf, 1947, 1951).

13. Leonard, footnote 1 (this chapter), pp. 9–10. By permission of Delacorte Press.

14. Hal Lindsey, *The Late, Great Planet Earth* (New York: Bantam Books, 1973).

15. William Irwin Thompson, "Planetary Vistas," *Harpers,* **243** (December 1971), 73.

16. Daniel Yankelovich, "The New Naturalism," *Saturday Review,* **55** (April 1972), 35. Copyright 1972 by Saturday Review Co. First appeared in *Saturday Review,* April 1972. Used with permission of the author and the publisher.

17. See footnote 50, Chapter 4.

18. See, for example, Thomas R. Brendle and Claude W. Unger, *Folk Medicine of the Pennsylvania Germans, The Non-Occult Cures* (Clifton, N.J.: Augustus M. Kelley, 1970).

19. W. W. Bauer, M.D., addresses this issue in *Potions, Remedies and Old Wives Tales* (Garden City, N.Y.: Doubleday, 1969).

20. See footnote 22, Chapter 3.

21. Andrew Weil, M.D., *The Natural Mind* (Boston: Houghton Mifflin, 1972).

22. *Ibid.*, p. 137.

23. *Ibid.*, p. 161. See also Neal E. Miller, "Learning of Visceral and Glandular Responses," *Science,* **163** (1969), 434–448.

24. See the discussion of biofeedback in Chapter 3.

25. The number of books and articles on the subject is staggering. Among them the following are noteworthy: Willis Harmon, "The New Copernican Revolution," *Stanford Today,* Winter 1969; Gopi Krishna, "Beyond the Higher States of Consciousness," *The New York Times,* October 6, 1973; and O. W. Markley et al., *Changing Images of Man,* Stanford Research Institute, October 1973. A compendium of works can be found in Michael Marien, "The Psychic Frontier: Toward New Paradigms for Man," *The World Institute Guide to Alternative Futures for Health* (New York: World Institute Council, n.d.).

26. Robert S. DeRopp, *The Master Game* (New York: Dell Publishing Company, 1968).

27. *Ibid.*, p. 50.

28. William James, *The Varieties of Religious Experience* (New York: Longmans, Green and Co., 1929), p. 388.

29. See, for example, footnotes 46 and 51, Chapter 3. See also Lawrence LeShan, *The Medium, the Mystic and the Physicist* (New York: Viking Press, 1974).

30. There are two books worth noting here, although neither fully develops the implications of expanded levels of consciousness for health. They are Robert Ornstein, *The Psychology of Consciousness* (New York: Viking Press, 1972), and Claudio Naranjo, *The One Quest* (New York: Viking Press, 1972).

31. Barry Commoner, *The Closing Circle* (New York: Knopf, 1971), p. 18. © 1971 by Barry Commoner. By permission of Alfred A. Knopf, Inc.

32. *Ibid.*, p. 18.

33. Theobald, footnote 7 (this chapter), p. 1.

34. Kenneth Boulding, "Ecology and Environment," *Trans-action,* March 1970, 38.

35. Jacques Ellul, *The Technological Society* (New York: Vintage Books, 1964).

36. Carlos Castaneda, *The Teachings of Don Juan: A Yaqui Way of Knowledge* (Berkeley: University of California Press and Ballantine Books, 1968), pp. 91–94. Originally published by the University of California Press; reprinted by permission of The Regents of the University of California.

37. Theodore Roszak, *Where the Wasteland Ends* (Garden City, N.Y.: Doubleday, 1972).

38. Weil, footnote 21 (this chapter), p. 140.

39. The episode is recounted in Arthur Koestler, *The Roots of Coincidence* (New York: Random House, 1972), pp. 91–92. © 1972 by Arthur Koestler. By permission of Random House, Inc.

40. Sheila Ostrander and Lynn Schroeder, *Psychic Discoveries Behind the Iron Curtain* (Englewood Cliffs, N.J.: Prentice-Hall, 1970).

41. Koestler, footnote 39, this chapter.

42. Two general references for the subject are A. Argoff and Betty Shapin (eds.), *Parapsychology Today: A Geographic View* (New York: Parapsychology Foundation, 1973), and Milan Ryzl, *Parapsychology: A Scientific Approach* (New York: Hawthorn Books, 1970).

43. Koestler, footnote 39 (this chapter), pp. 47–48. © by Arthur Koestler. By permission of Random House, Inc.

44. This is a paraphrase of Koestler's account of Walter's experiment. See Koestler, footnote 39 (this chapter), pp. 123–124.

45. Andrija Puharich, *Beyond Telepathy* (Garden City, N.Y.: Doubleday Anchor Books, 1973).

46. Andrija Puharich, *Uri* (Garden City, N.Y.: Doubleday, 1974).

47. See, for example, *Time,* March 4, 1974.

48. Russel Targ and Harold Puthoff, "Information Transmission Under Conditions of Sensory Shielding," *Nature,* **251** (October 18, 1974), 602–607.

49. Unpublished report of the Stanford Research Institute, 1973.

50. Koestler, footnote 39 (this chapter), p. 53.

51. A recent attempt to develop a theory of the paranormal is contained in a book by Larry LeShan, footnote 30, this chapter.

52. See Ostrander and Schroeder, footnote 40, this chapter.

53. Harold S. Burr, *The Fields of Life: Our Links With the Universe* (London: Neville Spearman, Ltd., 1971).

54. See Cleve Backster, "Evidence of Primary Perception in Plant Life," *International Journal of Parapsychology,* **10** (1968), 4.

55. The work of Cleve Backster has been reported in a number of publications. See, for example, Lyall Watson, *Supernature* (Garden City, N.Y.: Doubleday Anchor Books, 1973). On the subject in general, see also E. Stanton Maxey, M.D., "Man, Mind, Matter and Fields," unpublished paper, May Lecture Proceedings, London, May 1974.

56. Maxey, footnote 55, this chapter.

57. Michael Gauquelin, *The Cosmic Clocks* (London: Peter Owen, 1969). See also his *The Scientific Basis of Astrology* (New York: Stein & Day, 1969).

58. Gunther Stent, "Prematurity and Uniqueness in Scientific Discovery," *Scientific American,* **227** (December 1972), 84–93.

59. Watson, footnote 55, this chapter.

60. *Ibid.,* pp. viii–ix.

61. *Ibid.,* pp. 307–308.

62. *Ibid.,* p. 179.

63. See, for example, research reported by Danish researchers in *New Scientist,* November 8, 1973. There is other research on specific wave functions. For example, see H. Kenig, "Biological Effects of Extremely Low Frequency Electrical Phenomena in Atmosphere," *Journal of Interdisciplinary Cycle Research,* **12,** 3; and H. H. Heller, "Cellular Effects of Microwave Radiation," Symposium proceedings, Richmond, Va., September 1969.

64. This anecdote is also recorded in Watson's *Supernature,* footnote 55, this chapter.

65. John Ott, *Health and Light* (Old Greenwich, Conn.: Devin-Adair, 1973).

66. *Ibid.,* pp. 105–106. Copyright 1973 by John Ott Pictures, Inc. By permission of the Devin-Adair Co., Old Greenwich, Conn., publishers.

67. Christopher Jencks et al., *Inequality* (New York: Basic Books, 1972).

68. Ivan D. Illich, *Deschooling Society* (New York: Harper & Row, 1970).

69. Ivan D. Illich, *Tools for Conviviality* (New York: Harper & Row, 1973).

70. *Ibid.,* p. 7. By permission of Harper & Row.

71. The outlines of this analysis are owed to Ivan Illich in his essay, "The Political Uses of Death," *Hastings Center Studies,* **2,** 1 (January 1974).

72. Of course, shamans also performed "cures" in less "terminal" cases. And in this sense, their role was closer to that of the modern physician.

73. Elisabeth Kübler-Ross, M.D., *On Death and Dying* (New York: Macmillan, 1969).

CHAPTER 6

1. A good, brief account of their work can be found in Robert S. De-Ropp, *The New Prometheans* (New York: Dell Publishing Company, 1972).

2. See, for example, Aaron Antolnovsky, "Breakdown. A Needed Armamentarium of Modern Medicine," *Social Science and Medicine,* **6** (1972), 537–544.

3. For a discussion of "sick roles," see Miriam Siegler and Humphrey Osmond, "The Sick Role Revisited," *Hastings Center Studies,* **1,** 3, 41.

4. René Dubos, *Man Adapting* (New Haven: Yale University Press, 1965), p. 346.

5. Gregory Bateson, *Steps to an Ecology of Mind* (New York: Ballantine Books, 1972), p. 493.

6. Mike Samuels, M.D., and Hal Bennett, *The Well Body Book* (New York: Random House and The Bookworks, 1973).

7. Roszak, footnote 37 (Chapter 5), p. 99.

8. Gay Gaer Luce, *Body Time: Physiological Rhythms and Social Issues* (New York: Pantheon, 1971).

9. *Ibid.,* pp. viii–ix. © 1971, by Gay Gaer Luce. By permission of Pantheon Books/A Division of Random House, Inc.

10. These data are drawn from Fuchs, "Some Economic Aspects of Mortality in Developed Countries" (see footnote 56, Chapter 2).

11. Other factors probably include better overall health on the part of those who marry and the regularity of the lives of married men.

12. Sören Kierkegaard, *Fear and Trembling* (Garden City, N.Y.: Doubleday, 1954), pp. 49–52.

13. See *Time,* March 18, 1974.

14. Roger J. Williams, "You Are Biochemically Unique," *Intellectual Digest,* April 1974, 52.

15. See John McHale, *The Ecological Context* (New York: George Braziller, 1970). McHale says, "Though seemingly innocuous in its theoretical origins, ecology generates a radical view of human society, which may prove to be more 'positively' revolutionary . . . than any of the socio-political ideologies" (p. 1).

16. Captain Bob Hoke, "Health and Healthing: Beyond Disease and Dysfunctional Environments," paper presented at the Annual Meeting of the American Association for the Advancement of Science, Washington, D.C., December 30, 1972. See also his "Man-Environment Relations and Healing," paper prepared for the American Psychiatric Association Annual Meeting, Honolulu, Hawaii, 1973.

17. John Dewey and A. F. Bentley, *Knowing and the Known* (Boston: Beacon Press, 1960).

18. Fredrick Sargent III, "Man-Environment Problems for Public Health," *American Journal of Public Health,* **62,** 5 (1972), 626–633.

19. Captain Bob Hoke, "Promotive Medicine and the Phenomenon of Health," *Archives of Environmental Health,* **16,** 269–278.

20. Marc LaLonde, Minister of National Health and Welfare, *A New Perspective on the Health of Canadians* (Ottawa: Government of Canada, 1974), pp. 5–6.

21. See *Disease, Life and Man, Selected Essays by Rudolf Virchow,* Helfand Rather (trans.) (Stanford: Stanford University Press, 1958).

CHAPTER 7

1. See, for example, H. Sigerist, *Civilization and Disease* (Ithaca, N.Y.: Cornell University Press, 1943), where the author traces the interconnections between medicine and society.

2. Eliot Freidson, *Profession of Medicine* (New York: Dodd, Head, 1970), p. 251 (emphasis in original).

3. Garrett Hardin, "The Tragedy of the Commons," *Science*, **162** (December 13, 1968), 1243–1248.

4. The fact that providers of medical care do stimulate a demand for their services is incontrovertible. See, for example, U.S. Department of Health, Education, and Welfare, "Determinants of Expenditure for Physicians' Services in the U.S., 1948–1968," DHEW Pub. no. 73-3013, December 1972. See also John P. Bunker, "Surgical Manpower," *New England Journal of Medicine*, **282**, 3 (January 15, 1970).

5. There are some doubters; among them is Harry Schwartz, who argues that the worst of the cost crunch is over. See Harry Schwartz, *The Case for American Medicine: A Realistic Look at Our Health Care System* (New York: David McKay Co., 1972).

6. This analysis does not take into consideration earlier "medicines," such as Greek or Roman medicine. Greek medicine was quite "scientific." I start the analysis roughly in the Dark Ages.

7. Jerome Frank, *Persuasion and Healing* (New York: Schocken Books, 1961).

8. Lord Ritchie-Calder, *Medicine and Man* (New York: Signet Science Library, 1958), p. 13.

9. Quoted in Frank, footnote 7 (this chapter), p. 65. Copyright 1961 by The Johns Hopkins University Press. Used by permission of Johns Hopkins University Press.

10. See John Powles, "On the Limitations of Modern Medicine," *Science, Medicine and Man*, **1** (1973), 13. Headington Hill Hall, Oxford, England: Pergamon Press, Ltd. Used by permission of Pergamon Press, Ltd.

11. Rudolf Virchow, *Cellular Pathology*, Frank Chance (trans.) (Ann Arbor, Mich.: Edwards Bros., 1940).

12. See DeRopp, footnote 26, Chapter 5.

13. See Max von Pettenkofer, "The Value of Health to a City," lectures quoted in *Bulletin of the History of Medicine*, **10** (1941), 487–503.

14. René Dubos, *So Human an Animal* (New York: Charles Scribner's Sons, 1968), pp. 227–229. Reprinted by permission of Charles Scribner's Sons. Copyright © 1968 René Dubos.

15. See footnote 59, Chapter 3, and footnote 55, Chapter 5. There are numerous anecdotal accounts of the Philippine practice. My comments are based on observations reported to me by Lyall Watson.

16. This point is developed in some detail in Chapter 4. See also, A. L. Cochrane, *Effectiveness and Efficiency* (London: The Nuffield Provincial Hospitals Trust, 1972).

17. It may be gaining in respectability. Authoritative commentators like Jerome Frank are beginning to assess its importance. See Frank, "The Gift of Healing: Is It Myth or Measurable Fact?" *Hospital Physician,* January 1974.

18. Claude Bernard, *An Introduction to Experimental Medicine,* H. C. Greene (trans.) (New York: Macmillan, 1927).

19. This view has contemporary adherents. See, for example, Aubrey T. Westlake, M.D., *The Pattern of Health* (Berkeley: Shambala Publications, 1973).

20. Abraham Flexner, *Medical Education in the United States and Canada* (New York: Carnegie Foundation for the Advancement of Teaching, 1910).

21. A. C. Crombie, "The Future of Biology, the History of a Program," *Federal Procedure,* **25** (1966), 1448–1453.

22. Powles, footnote 10 (this chapter), p. 15. Headington Hill Hall, Oxford, England: Pergamon Press, Ltd. Used by permission of Pergamon Press, Ltd.

23. *Ibid.,* p. 19.

24. Leo Tolstoy, "The Death of Ivan Illyich," in *Leo Tolstoi, Short Stories,* Margaret Wettlin (trans.) Moscow: Progress Publishers, n.d., pp. 108–167.

25. Schwartz, footnote 5, this chapter.

26. For a general description of the "health maintenance organization," see Paul M. Ellwood, Jr. et al., "Health Maintenance Strategy," *Medical Care,* **9,** 3 (May/June 1971).

27. Barbara Ehrenreich and John Ehrenreich, *The American Health Empire: Power, Profits and Politics* (New York: Random House, 1970). © 1970 by Health Policy Advisory Center, Inc. By permission of Random House, Inc.

28. *Ibid.,* p. 117.

29. *The Los Angeles Times,* August 26, 1973. See also Greer Williams, "Quality vs. Quantity in American Medical Education," *Science,* **153** (August 26, 1966).

30. Rashi Fein, "On Achieving Access and Equity in Health Care," *Milbank Memorial Fund Quarterly,* **50,** 4 (October, 1972), 158–159. By permission of the Milbank Memorial Fund.

31. Jerome Schwartz, "A Critical Review and Evaluation of Smoking Control Methods," *Public Health Report,* **84,** 6 (June 1969).

32. An argument that this is the medicine we need is offered by Michael De Bakey, M.D., in an article in *Saturday Review/World,* "Medical Prognosis: Favorable, Treatable, Curable," (Aug. 1974), pp. 46–48.

33. The research was reviewed in *The Los Angeles Times,* November 14, 1973 (emphasis added). Some earlier findings can be found in Lester Breslow and Bonnie Klein, "Health and Race in California," *American Journal of Public Health,* **61,** 4 (April 1971).

34. Although I do not entirely relish the association, the best piece on this subject I have read is a chapter by Milton Friedman in his book, *Capitalism and Freedom* (Chicago: University of Chicago Press, 1962).

35. See Sister Justa Smith, Ph.D., "Paranormal Effects on Enzyme Activity," *Human Dimensions,* **1,** 2 (Spring 1972).

36. John Radar Platt, "Hierarchical Restructuring," *Bulletin of Atomic Scientists,* November 1970.

37. Ivan D. Illich, *Celebration of Awareness* (Garden City, N.Y.: Doubleday, 1970), p. 163.

38. Peter Sedgewick, "Illness—Mental and Otherwise," *Hastings Center Studies,* **3** (1973), 37.

EPILOGUE

1. As Chapter 2 indicates, the technology of outcomes assessment must be rapidly improved if this is to be accomplished.

2. For a fascinating article on the relationship between disease and old age, see Alexander Leaf, M.D., "Three Score and Forty," *Hospital Practice,* October 1973, reprinted in *Intellectual Digest,* March 1974.

Bibliography

Abey-Wickrama, I., et al. "Mental Hospital Admissions and Aircraft Noise," *The Lancet,* December 13, 1969.

Abel-Smith, Brian. *An International Study of Health Expenditures.* Geneva: World Health Organization, 1967.

Alexander, F. M. *The Use of Self.* Manchester: Re-educational Publications, Ltd., 1932.

Alexander, Rolf. *Creative Realism.* New York: Pageant Press, 1954.

Anderson, Odin W. *Health Care: Can There Be Equity?* New York: Wiley-Interscience, 1973.

Andervont, H. B. "Influences of Environment on Mammary Cancer in Mice," *Journal of the National Cancer Institute,* **4** (1964).

Anticaglia, Joseph R., and Cohen, Alexander. "Extra-Auditory Effects of Noise as a Health Hazard," *American Industrial Hygiene Association Journal,* **31** (1970).

Antolnovsky, Aaron. "Breakdown: A Needed Armamentarium of Modern Medicine," *Social Science and Medicine,* **6** (1972).

Argoff, A., and Shapin, Betty, eds. *Parapsychology Today: A Geographic View.* New York: Parapsychology Foundation, 1973.

Audy, J. Ralph, M.D. "Man-Made Maladies and Medicine," *California Medicine,* November, 1970.

Auster, Richard; Levison, Irving; and Sarachek, Deborah. "The Production of Health; An Exploratory Study," *Journal of Human Resources,* **4,** 4 (Fall 1969).

Backster, Cleve. "Evidence of Primary Perception in Plant Life," *International Journal of Parapsychology,* **10** (1968).

Barber, Theodore, et al., eds. *Biofeedback and Self-Control.* Chicago: Aldine Publishing Company, 1971.

Baron, Robert. *The Tyranny of Noise.* New York: St. Martin's Press, 1970.

Bateson, Gregory. *Steps to an Ecology of Mind.* New York: Ballantine Books, 1972.

Bauer, W. W., M.D. *Potions, Remedies and Old Wives Tales.* Garden City, N.Y.: Doubleday, 1969.

Bell, Daniel, ed. *Toward the Year 2000: Work in Progress.* Boston: Daedalus Library, Beacon Press, 1967–1968.

Bergman, A. B., and Stamm, S. J. "The Morbidity of Cardiac Non-Disease in Schoolchildren," *New England Journal of Medicine,* **276,** 18 (May 4, 1967).

Berk, J. Edward, M.D. "Major U.S. Ailment Receives Little Attention, Doctor Says," *The Los Angeles Times,* November 6, 1972.

Bernard, Claude. *An Introduction to Experimental Medicine.* H. C. Greene, trans. New York: Macmillan, 1927.

Blumgart, Herrman L. "Caring for the Patient," *New England Journal of Medicine,* **270** (1964), 449.

Boulding, Kenneth. "Ecology and Environment," *Trans-action,* March 1970.

Brecher, Edward M., and the Editors of *Consumer Reports. Licit and Illicit Drugs.* Mount Vernon, N.Y.: Consumers Union, 1972.

Brena, Steven, M.D. *Yoga and Medicine.* New York: Julian Press, Inc., 1972.

Brendle, Thomas R., and Unger, Claude W. *Folk Medicine of the Pennsylvania Germans, The Non-Occult Cures.* Clifton, N.J.: Augustus M. Kelley, 1970.

Breslow, Lester, and Klein, Bonnie. "Health and Race in California," *American Journal of Public Health,* **61,** 4 (April 1971).

Brockington, Colin Fraser. *World Health.* Baltimore: Penguin Books, 1958.

Brook, Robert H., M.D., Sc.D., et al. "Effectiveness of Non-Emergency Care via an Emergency Room," *Annals of Internal Medicine,* **78** (1973).

Brown, Barbara, *New Mind, New Body.* New York: Harper & Row, 1974.

Brown, G. W., and Birley, J. L. "Crises and Life Changes and the Onset of Schizophrenia," *Journal of Health and Social Behavior,* **9** (September 1968).

Bryant, John. *Health and the Developing World.* Ithaca, N.Y.: Cornell University Press, 1969.

Budzynski, Thomas H.; Stoyva, Johann; and Adler, Charles. "Feedback-Induced Muscle Relaxation: Application to Tension Headaches," *Journal of Behavioral Therapy and Experimental Psychology,* **1.**

Bunker, John P. "Surgical Manpower," *New England Journal of Medicine,* **282,** 3 (January 15, 1970).

Burr, Harold S. *The Fields of Life: Our Links With the Universe.* London: Neville Spearman, Ltd., 1971.

Caghill, G. E. "Appreciation: The Educational Methods of F. M. Alexander." In Alexander, F. M., *The Unusual Constant in Living.* New York: Dutton, 1941.

Calder, Lord Ritchie. *Medicine and Man.* New York: Signet Science Library, 1958.

Calhoun, J. B. "Population Density and Social Pathology," *Scientific American,* **206** (1962).

California State Department of Public Health, Senate Committee. "Fatal

Aplastic Anemia in California, Its Relationship to the Drug Chloramphenicol." November 23, 1962.

Carson, Rachel. *Silent Spring*. Boston: Houghton Mifflin, 1962.

Cassel, John C., M.D. "Health Consequences of Population and Crowding." A paper presented at the American Medical Association Congress on Environmental Health, Los Angeles, April 24–25, 1972. "Epidemiology and Mental Health" in *Mental Health Considerations in Public Health,* Public Health Service Publication 1898 (Washington, D.C., Government Printing Office, May, 1969), p. 67.

Castaneda, Carlos. *A Separate Reality*. New York: Simon & Schuster, 1971.

———. *The Teachings of Don Juan: A Yaqui Way of Knowledge*. Berkeley: University of California Press and Ballantine Books, 1968.

Chase, Allen. *The Biological Imperatives*. New York: Holt, Rinehart and Winston, 1972.

Chicago Hospital Council. "The Crisis in Emergency Care, Part 1. The Ambulance Scandal: A Hazard to Life and Health," *Medical World News,* **11** (December 4, 1970).

Cochrane, A. L., CBE, FREP. *Effectiveness and Efficiency*. London: The Nuffield Provincial Hospitals Trust, 1972.

Codman, E. A. "The Product of the Hospital," *Surgery, Gynecology and Obstetrics,* **18** (1914).

Coles, Robert. "The Case of Michael Wechsler," *New York Review of Books,* May 18, 1972.

Comfort, Alexander. *The Process of Aging*. London: Weidenfelt & Nicholson, 1964.

Committee of Public Health. "Air Pollution and Health," *The New York Adademy of Medicine Bulletin,* **42,** 7 (July 1966).

Committee on Environmental Hazards of the American Academy of Pediatricians. "Acute and Chronic Childhood Lead Poisoning," *Pediatrics,* **47,** 5 (May 1971).

Commoner, Barry. *The Closing Circle*. New York: Knopf, 1971.

———. "Workplace Burden," *Environment,* July/August 1973.

Cooper, Brian; Fry, John; and Kalton, Graham. "A Longitudinal Study of Psychiatric Morbidity in a General Practice Population," *British Journal of Preventive and Social Medicine,* **23** (1969).

Crombie, A. C. "The Future of Biology, the History of a Program," *Federal Procedures,* **25** (1966).

Cros, J. F. "Chemical Risk to Future Generations," *Scientist and Citizen,* **10** (1968).

Dart, R. A. "An Anatomist's Tribute to F. M. Alexander," *South Africa Medical Journal,* **21** (1947).

De Bakey, Michael, M.D. "Medical Prognosis: Favorable, Treatable, Curable," *Saturday Review/World,* Aug. 24, 1974, pp. 46–48.

DeBrigard, Raul, and Helmer, Olaf. "Some Potential Societal Developments, 1970–2000." Report of Research, The Institute for the Future, IFF Report R–7, 1970.

DeRopp, Robert S. *The Master Game.* New York: Dell Publishing Company, 1968.

———. *The New Prometheans.* New York: Dell Publishing Company, 1972.

Dewey, John, and Bentley, A. F. *Knowing and the Known.* Boston: Beacon Press, 1960.

DiCara, Leo V. "Learning in the Autonomic Nervous System," *Scientific American,* January 1970.

Dimensions of Healing: A Symposium. The American Academy of Parapsychology and Medicine, San Francisco, 1973.

Dohrenwend, Bruce P., and Dohrenwend, Barbara S. *Social Status and Psychological Disorder: A Causal Inquiry.* New York: Wiley-Interscience, 1969.

Doxiadis, Constantine, "Confessions of a Criminal," *Los Angeles Times,* January 7, 1973.

Doyle, James C. "Unnecessary Hysterectomies: Study of 6,248 Operations in 35 Hospitals in 1948," *Journal of the American Medical Association,* **151** (1963).

———. "Unnecessary Ovariectomies," *Journal of the American Medical Association,* **148,** 13 (1952).

Drucker, Peter. "The New Markets and the New Capitalism," *The Public Interest,* Fall 1970.

Dubos, René. *Man Adapting.* New Haven: Yale University Press, 1965.

———. *Man, Medicine and Environment.* New York: Praeger, 1968.

———. *Mirage of Health.* New York: World Perspectives, Harper & Row, 1959.

———. "Promises and Hazards of Man's Adaptability." In Jarrett, Henry, ed., *Environmental Quality in a Growing Economy.* Baltimore: The Johns Hopkins University Press, 1966.

———. *So Human an Animal.* New York: Charles Scribner's Sons, 1968.

———. *White Plague: Tuberculosis, Man and Society.* Boston: Little, Brown, 1952.

Dumont, Matthew, M.D. *The Absurd Healer.* New York: Viking Press, 1971.

Ehrenreich, Barbara, and Ehrenreich, John. *The American Health Empire: Power, Profits and Politics.* New York: Random House, 1970.

Ellul, Jacques. *The Technological Society.* New York: Vintage Books, 1964.

Ellwood, Paul M., Jr., et al. "Health Maintenance Strategy," *Medical Care,* **9,** 3 (May/June 1971).

Epstein, Samuel S., and Legator, Marvin S., eds. *The Mutagenicity of Pesticides: Concepts and Evaluation.* Cambridge: The MIT Press, 1971.

Erikson, Kai T. *Wayward Pilgrims.* New York: John Wiley & Sons, 1966.

Etzioni, Amitai. *Genetic Fix: New Opportunities and Dangers for You, Your Child and the Nation.* New York: Macmillan, 1973.

Evans, Frederick. "The Power of a Sugar Pill," *Psychology Today,* April 1974.

Evans, H. E. "Tonsillectomy and Adenoidectomy: Review of Published Evidence For and Against T. and A.," *Clinical Pediatrics,* **7** (1968).

Eversa, T. D., and Cole, W. H. *Spontaneous Regression of Cancer.* Philadelphia: W. B. Saunders Co., 1966.

Fein, Rashi. "On Achieving Access and Equity in Health Care," *Milbank Memorial Fund Quarterly,* **50,** 4 (October 1972).

Flexner, Abraham. *Medical Education in the United States and Canada.* New York: Carnegie Foundation for the Advancement of Teaching, 1910.

Folgyesi, F. A. "School for Patients," *British Journal of Medical Hypnotism,* **5** (1954).

Folile, E. W., and Marches, J. E. "Mental Health Morbidity in a Suburban Community," *Journal of Clinical Psychology,* **24,** 1 (1968).

Forrester, Jay. *World Dynamics.* Cambridge: Wright-Allen Press, 1971.

Frank, Jerome. "The Gift of Healing: Is It Myth or Measurable Fact?" *Hospital Physician,* January 1974.

———. *Persuasion and Healing.* New York: Schocken Books, 1961.

Freedland, N. *The Occult Explosion.* London: Michael Joseph, 1972.

Freese, Arthur. "Trauma: The Neglected Epidemic," *Saturday Review,* May 13, 1972.

Freidson, Eliot. *Professional Dominance.* New York: Atherton Press, 1971.

———. "Professionalism: The Doctor's Dilemma," *Social Policy,* January/February, 1971.

———. *Profession of Medicine.* New York: Dodd, Mead, 1970.

Friedenburg, Edgar Z. *Laing.* New York: Viking Press, 1974.

Friedman, Milton. *Capitalism and Freedom.* Chicago: University of Chicago Press, 1962.

Fuchs, Victor. "The Contribution of Health Services to the American Economy," *Milbank Memorial Fund Quarterly,* **44,** 4 (October 1966).

———. *The Service Economy.* New York: National Bureau of Economic Research, 1968.

———. "Some Economic Aspects of Mortality in Developed Countries." A paper presented to the International Economic Association Conference on Economics of Health and Medical Care, Tokyo, April 2–7, 1973.

Fuller, John G. *Arigo: Surgeon of the Rusty Knife.* New York: Thomas Y. Crowell, 1974.

Gauquelin, Michael. *The Cosmic Clocks.* London: Peter Owen, 1969.

———. *The Scientific Basis of Astrology.* New York: Stein & Day, 1969.

Ginzberg, Eli. *Men, Money, and Medicine.* New York: Columbia University Press, 1969.

Goble, Frank. *The Third Force.* New York: Grossman Publishers, 1970.

Goldhammer, Herbert, and Marshall, Andrew. *Psychosis and Civilization.* Glencoe, Ill.: The Free Press, 1949.

Gordon, J. B.; Ahman, A.; and Brodis, M. C. *Industrial Safety Statistics: A Re-Examination.* New York: Praeger, 1971.

Grant, Neville, M.D. "Mercury in Man," *Environment,* **13** (May 1971).

Green, Elmer E. "Biofeedback for Mind-Body Self-Regulation: Healing and Creativity." In *The Varieties of Healing Experience.* Transcript of the Interdisciplinary Symposium of the American Academy of Parapsychology and Medicine, San Francisco, October 30, 1971.

————. "How to Make Use of the Field of Mind Theory." In *Dimensions of Healing: A Symposium.* The American Academy of Parapsychology and Medicine, San Francisco, 1973.

Greenblatt, M.; Emery, P.; and Glueck, B. *Poverty and Mental Health.* Psychiatric Research Report no. 22. Washington, D.C. American Psychiatric Association, 1967.

Grier, George. *The Changing Age Profile, Implications for Policy Planning in Metropolitan Washington.* Washington, D.C.: Washington Center for Metropolitan Studies, 1964.

Grosse, Robert N. "Cost-Benefit Analysis of Health Services," *The Annals of the American Academy of Political and Social Science,* **399** (January 1972).

Hamilton, Michael P., ed. *The New Genetics of the Future of Man.* Grand Rapids, Mich.: Eerdmans Publishing Co,, 1972.

Hammond, E. C., and Horn, D. "Smoking and Death Rates: Report on Forty-four Months of Follow-up of 186,763 Men," *Journal of the American Medical Association,* **166** (1958).

Hampden-Turner, Charles. *Radical Man.* Cambridge: Schenkman Publishing Co., 1970.

Handler, Seymour, M.D. "Bring Back the Mustard Plaster," *Minnesota Medicine,* **54** (December 1971).

Hardin, Garrett. "The Tragedy of the Commons," *Science,* **162** (December 13, 1968).

Harmon, Willis. "The New Copernican Revolution," *Stanford Today,* Winter 1969.

Heller, H. H. "Cellular Effects of Microwave Radiation," Symposium proceedings, Richmond, Va., September 1969.

Hoke, Captain Bob. "Health and Healthing: Beyond Disease and Dysfunctional Environments." A paper presented at the Annual Meeting of the American Association for the Advancement of Science, Washington, D.C., December 30, 1972.

————. "Man-Environment Relations and Healing." A paper prepared for the American Psychiatric Association Annual Meeting, Honolulu, Hawaii, 1973.

———. "Promotive Medicine and the Phenomenon of Health," *Archives of Environmental Health,* **16.**

Hollingshead, A. B., and Redlich, F. C., *Social Class and Mental Illness.* New York: John Wiley & Sons, Inc., 1958.

Holmes, J. H., and Masuda, M. "Psychosomatic Syndrome," *Psychology Today,* April 1972.

Holmes, Oliver Wendell, Sr. *Medical Essays.* Boston: Houghton Mifflin, 1907.

Horn, Joshua S. *Away With All Pests.* New York: Modern Reader Paperback, 1971.

Horton, P. B., and Leslie, G. K. *The Sociology of Social Problems.* New York: Appleton-Century-Crofts, 1965.

Hurley, Rodger L. *Poverty and Mental Retardation.* New York: Random House, 1969.

Illich, Ivan D. *Celebration of Awareness.* Garden City, N.Y.: Doubleday, 1970.

———. *Deschooling Society.* New York: Harper & Row, 1970.

———. *Medical Nemesis.* London: Calder and Boyars, 1974.

———. "The Political Uses of Death," *Hastings Center Studies,* **2,** 1 (January 1974).

———. *Tools for Conviviality.* New York: Harper & Row, 1973.

James, William. *The Varieties of Religious Experience.* New York: Longmans, Green and Co., 1929.

Jencks, Christopher, et al. *Inequality.* New York: Basic Books, 1972.

Kahn, Herman, and Wiener, A. J. *The Year 2000: A Framework for Speculation on the Next Thirty-Three Years.* New York: Macmillan, 1967.

Karagula, Shafica, M.D. *Breakthrough to Creativity.* Los Angeles: DeVorss and Co., Inc., 1967.

Kasl, Stanley V., Ph.D.; Cobb, Sidney, M.D.; and Brooks, George W., M.P.H. "Changes in Serum Uric Acid and Cholesterol Levels in Men Undergoing Job Loss," *Journal of the American Medical Association,* **206,** 7 (November 11, 1968).

Kasl, Stanley V., and Cobb, Sidney. "Effects of Parental Status Incongruence and Discrepancy on Physical and Mental Health of Adult Offspring," *Journal of Personality and Social Psychology,* **7,** 2 (October 1967).

Kenig, H. "Biological Effects of Extremely Low Frequency Electrical Phenomenon in Atmosphere," *Journal of Interdisciplinary Cycle Research,* **12,** 3.

Kessner, David, M.D. Unpublished report of the Institute of Medicine, National Academy of Sciences, n.d.

Kierkegaard, Sören. *Fear and Trembling.* Garden City, N.Y.: Doubleday, 1954.

Klebba, A. J. "Mortality Trends in the U.S. 1954–1963," publ. 1000, ser. 20, no. 2. Washington, D.C.: Public Health Service, 1965.

Klerman, Gerald L. "Psychotropic Drugs as Therapeutic Agents," *Hastings Center Studies*, **2**, 1 (January 1974).

Koenig, Peter. "The Placebo Effect in Patent Medicine," *Psychology Today*, April 1973.

Koestler, Arthur. *The Ghost in the Machine*. New York: Macmillan, 1968.

————. *The Roots of Coincidence*. New York: Random House, 1972.

Krippner, S., and Rubin, D., eds. *Galaxies of Life: The Human Aura in Acupuncture and Kirlian Photography*. New York: Gordon and Breach, 1973.

Krishna, Gopi. "Beyond the Higher States of Consciousness," *New York Times,* October 6, 1973.

Kübler-Ross, Elisabeth, M.D. *On Death and Dying*. New York: Macmillan, 1969.

Kuhn, Thomas. *The Structure of Scientific Revolutions*. Chicago: University of Chicago Press, 1962.

Laing, R. D. *The Politics of Experience*. New York: Ballantine, 1970.

LaLonde, Marc, Minister of National Health and Welfare, The Government of Canada. *A New Perspective on the Health of Canadians*. Ottawa: Government of Canada, 1974.

Landsberger, Henry A. *Hawthorne Revisited*. Ithaca, N.Y.: Cornell University Press, 1958.

"Last Year at Deauville," *Environment,* **13** (July/August 1971).

Lave, L. B., and Seskin, E. P. "Air Pollution and Human Health," *Science,* **169,** 3947 (August 21, 1970).

Leaf, Alexander, M.D. "Three Score and Forty," *Hospital Practice,* October 1973.

Lefcowitz, Myron J. "Poverty and Health: A Reexamination," *Inquiry,* **10** (March 1973).

Lemkau, P.; Tietze, C.; and Cooper, M. *Mental Hygiene in Public Health*. New York: McGraw-Hill, 1949.

Leonard, George. *The Transformation: A Guide to the Inevitable Changes in Humankind*. New York: Delacorte Press, 1972.

LeShan, Lawrence. *The Medium, the Mystic and the Physicist*. New York: Viking Press, 1974.

Lewis, C. E. "Variations in Incidence of Surgery," *New England Journal of Medicine,* **281,** 6 (October 16, 1969).

Lewis, H. R., and Lewis, M. E. *Psychosomatics*. New York: Viking Press, 1972.

Liang, M. H., et al. "Chinese Health Care: Determinants of the System," *American Journal of Public Health,* **63,** 2 (February 1973).

Lin, Paul T. K. "Medicine in China," *The Center Magazine,* May/June 1974.

Lindsey, Hal. *The Late, Great Planet Earth*. New York: Bantam Books, 1973.

Lipton, Samuel D. "On Psychology of Childhood Tonsillectomy," *Psychoanalytic Study of the Child,* **17** (1962).

Looney, Gerald L. "Getting What We Pay For." A paper presented at the Third Annual Meeting of the Comprehensive Health Planning Council of Maricopa County, Phoenix, Arizona, November 19, 1971.

Lorenz, Konrad. *Civilized Man's Eight Deadly Sins.* New York: Harcourt Brace Jovanovich, 1974.

Luce, Gay Gaer. *Body Time: Physiological Rhythms and Social Issues.* New York: Pantheon, 1971.

Lynch, Henry, M.D., ed. *Cancer and You.* Springfield, Ill.: Charles C Thomas, 1971.

Maddox, John. *The Doomsday Syndrome.* New York: McGraw-Hill, 1972.

Marien, Michael. "The Psychic Frontier: Toward New Paradigms for Man," *The World Institute Guide to Alternative Futures for Health.* New York: World Institute Council, n.d.

Markley, O. W., et al. *Changing Images of Man.* Stanford Research Institute, October 1973.

Maslow, Abraham. *Toward a Psychology of Being.* New York: Van Nostrand, 1962.

Mather, H. G., et al. "Acute Myocardial Infarction: Home and Hospital Treatment," *British Medical Journal,* **3** (1971).

Matson, Floyd W. *The Broken Image.* Garden City, N.Y.: Doubleday, Anchor Books, 1966.

Maxey, E. Stanton, M.D. "Man, Mind, Matter and Fields," *The Frontiers of Science and Medicine,* ed. Rick J. Carlson, proceedings of a conf., London, 1974, in press, Wildwood House, 1975.

McCleery, Robert S., et al. *One Life—One Physician.* (New York: The Public Interest Press, 1971).

McDonald, J. Ross. "Radiation in Aircraft," *Environment,* **15** (July/August 1973).

McHale, John. *The Ecological Context.* New York: George Braziller, 1970.

McKeown, Thomas. *Time Trend Studies.* London: Oxford University Press and Nuffield Press, 1971.

Mechanic, David. "Health and Illness in Technological Societies," *Hastings Center Studies,* **1,** 3 (1973).

"Medical Manpower Specialty Distribution Projections: 1975 and 1980," Health Services Research Center Interstudy, Minneapolis, Minn., May 1971.

Melzack, Ronald. "How Acupuncture Works: A Sophisticated Western Theory Takes the Mystery Out," *Psychology Today,* June 1973.

Michaelson, Michael G. "The Failure of American Medicine," *The American Scholar,* **39,** 4 (Autumn 1970).

Miettinen, M., et al. "Effect of Cholesterol-Lowering Diet on Mortality from Coronary Heart Disease and Other Causes," *The Lancet,* **2** (October 21, 1972).

Miller, Neal E. "Learning of Visceral and Glandular Responses," *Science,* **163** (1969).

Moser, R. H. *Diseases of Medical Progress: A Study of Iatrogenic Disease,* 3d ed. Springfield, Ill.: Charles C Thomas, 1969.

Moses, Lincoln, and Mosteller, Frederick. "Institutional Differences in Post-Operative Death Rates," *Journal of the American Medical Association,* **162,** 7 (October 13, 1956).

Moss, Thelma, and Johnson, Kendall. "The Body is an Energy Field," *Harpers,* January 1973.

Muller, Charlotte. "The Over-Medicated Society: Forces in the Marketplace for Medical Care," *Science,* **176** (May 5, 1972).

Myrdal, Gunnar. *Asian Drama: An Inquiry into the Poverty of Nations.* New York: Vintage Books, 1971.

Naranjo, Claudio. *The One Quest.* New York: Viking Press, 1972.

National Center for Health Statistics. "Reports of the Division of Vital Statistics," Washington, D.C., 1967.

Newman, Oscar. *Architectural Design for Crime Prevention.* Washington, D.C.: National Institute of Law Enforcement and Criminal Justice, 1973.

Nobile, Philip. "King Cancer," *Esquire,* June 1973.

Ogra, Pearay L., M.D. "Effect of Tonsillectomy and Adenoidectomy on Nasopharyngeal Antibody Response to Poliovirus," *New England Journal of Medicine,* **284** (January 14, 1971).

Ornstein, Robert. *The Psychology of Consciousness.* New York: Viking Press, 1972.

Ostrander, Sheila, and Schroeder, Lynn. *Psychic Discoveries Behind the Iron Curtain.* Englewood Cliffs, N.J.: Prentice-Hall, 1970.

Ott, John. *Health and Light.* Old Greenwich, Conn.: Devin-Adair, 1973.

Pasamanick, B., ed. *Epidemiology of Mental Disorder.* Washington, D.C., American Association for the Advancement of Science, 1959.

Pekkanen, John. *The American Connection.* Chicago: Follett Publishing Co., 1973.

Pettenkofer, Max von. "The Value of Health to a City." Lectures quoted in *Bulletin of the History of Medicine,* **10** (1941).

Platt, John Radar. "Hierarchical Restructuring," *Bulletin of Atomic Scientists,* November 1970.

Powles, John. "On the Limitations of Modern Medicine," *Science, Medicine and Man,* **1** (1973).

Puharich, Andrija. *Beyond Telepathy.* Garden City, N.Y.: Doubleday Anchor Books, 1973.

————. *Uri.* Garden City, N.Y.: Doubleday Anchor Books, 1974.

Quinn, R. W., and Campbell, E. S. "Heart Disease in Children: Survey of School Children in Nashville, Tennessee," *Yale Journal of Biology and Medicine,* **34** (1962).

Rahe, Richard; McKean, Joseph, Jr.; and Arthur, Ransom. "A Longitudinal Study of Life Change and Illness Patterns," *Journal of Psychosomatic Research,* **10** 4 (1967).

Rauscher, Frank J. "Interview," *U.S. News and World Report,* December 4, 1972.

Rennie, Thomas A. C.; Srole, Leo; Opler, Marvin K.; and Langner, Thomas S. "Urban Life and Mental Health," *American Journal of Psychiatry,* **113** (157).

Ridken, Ronald. *Economic Costs of Air Pollution.* New York: Praeger, 1967.

Risley, Mary. *House of Healing: The Story of the Hospital.* Garden City, N.Y.: Doubleday, 1961.

Roemer, Milton I., M.D. *Medical Care in Relation to Public Health, A Monograph.* Geneva: World Health Organization, 1957.

Rosenham, Ray H., et al. "A Predictive Study of Coronary Heart Disease," *Journal of the American Medical Association,* **189** (1964).

Rosenhans, D. L. "On Being Sane in Insane Places," *Science,* **19** (January 19, 1973).

Roszak, Theodore. *Where the Wasteland Ends.* Garden City, N.Y.: Doubleday, 1972.

Rothman, David. *The Discovery of the Asylum.* Boston: Little, Brown, 1971.

Ryzl, Milan. *Parapsychology: A Scientific Approach.* New York: Hawthorne Books, 1970.

Salk, Jonas. *The Survival of the Wisest.* New York: Harper & Row, 1973.

Samuels, Mike, M.D., and Bennett, Hal. *The Well Body Book.* New York: Random House and The Bookworks, 1973.

Sargent, Fredrick, III. "Man-Environment Problems for Public Health," *American Journal of Public Health,* **62,** 5 (1972).

Sartre, Jean-Paul. *Roads to Freedom.* New York: Knopf, 1947, 1951.

Schoen, Donald. *Beyond the Stable State.* New York: Random House, 1971.

Schroeder, Harvey. "Metals in the Air," *Environment,* **13,** 8 (October 1971).

Schultz, Dodi. "The High Blood Pressure Time Bomb," *Viva,* April 1974.

Schwartz, Harry. *The Case for American Medicine: A Realistic Look at Our Health Care System.* New York: David McKay Co., 1972.

Schwartz, Jerome. "A Critical Review and Evaluation of Smoking Control Methods," *Public Health Report,* **84,** 6 (June 1969).

Sedgewick, Peter. "Illness—Mental and Otherwise," *Hastings Center Studies,* **3** (1973).

Segal, Ronald. *The Struggle Against History.* New York: Bantam Books, 1973.

Selye, Hans. *The Stress of Life.* New York: McGraw-Hill, 1956.

Shanas, Ethel. *The Health of Older People.* Cambridge: Harvard University Press, 1962.

Shapiro, A. K. "The Placebo Effect in the History of Medical Treatment: Implications for Psychiatry," *American Journal of Psychiatry,* **116** (1959).

Sherman, Harold. *Wonder Healers of the Philippines.* London: Psychic Press, 1967.

Shimkin, Demitri B. "Man, Ecology and Health," *Archives of Environmental Health,* **20** (January 1970).

Siegler, Miriam, and Osmond, Humphrey. "The Sick Role Revisited," *Hastings Center Studies,* **1,** 3.

Sigerist, H. *Civilization and Disease.* Ithaca, N.Y.: Cornell University Press, 1943.

Skinner, B. F. *Beyond Freedom and Dignity.* New York: Knopf, 1971.

Skipper, James K., Jr., and Leonard, Robert C. "Children, Stress and Hospitalizations: A Field Experiment," *Journal of Health and Social Behavior,* **9** (1968).

Smith, Sister Justa. "Paranormal Effects on Enzyme Activity," *Human Dimensions,* **1,** 2 (Spring 1972).

Somers, Anne. "Health Care and the Political System." A paper presented to the National Center for Health Service Research and Development Conference on Technology and Health Care Systems in the 1900s, Rockville, Maryland, January 19, 1972.

Srole, Leo; Lanner, Thomas S.; Michael, Stanley T.: Opler, Marvin K.; and Rennie, Thomas A. C. *Mental Health in the Metropolis: Midtown Manhattan Study.* New York: McGraw-Hill, 1962.

Srole, Leo; Langner, Thomas S.; and Rennie, Thomas A. C. "Mental Disorders in a Metropolis," *Public Health Report,* **72** (1963).

Starfield, Barbara, and Scheff, David. "Effectiveness of Pediatric Care: The Relationship Between Process and Outcome," *Pediatrics,* **49** (April 1972).

Stefansson, Vilhjalmur. *Cancer: Disease of Civilization.* New York: Hill & Wang, 1960.

Stent, Gunther. "Prematurity and Uniqueness in Scientific Discovery," *Scientific American,* **227** (December 1972).

Sterling, Theodore D. "Air Pollution and Smoking," *Environment,* July/August 1973.

Stewert, Charles T., Jr. "Allocation of Resources to Health," *Journal of Human Resources,* **6,** 2.

Stieglitz, Edward J. *The Second Forty Years.* Philadelphia: J. B. Lippincott Co., 1946.

Stocks, P. "On the Relations Between Atmospheric Pollution in Urban and Rural Localities and Mortality from Cancer, Bronchitis, and Pneumonia, with Particular Reference to 3, 4-Benayprene, Berylliu, Molybdenum, Vanadium, and Arsenic," *British Journal of Cancer*, **14** (1960).

Strickland, Stephen P. *Politics, Science, and Dread Disease.* Cambridge: Commonwealth Fund Book, Harvard University Press, 1972.

"A Study of Psychic Surgery and Spiritual Healing in the Philippines." Unpublished paper, July 1973.

Szasz, Thomas. *The Manufacture of Madness.* New York: Harper & Row, 1970.

Targ, Russel, and Puthoff, Harold. "Information Transmission Under Conditions of Sensory Shielding," *Nature*, **251** (October 18, 1974).

Taylor, Carl E., M.D., and Scrimshaw, Nevin. *Interactions of Nutrition and Infection.* Geneva: World Health Organization, 1968.

Taylor, Gordon Rattray. *The Biological Time Bomb.* New York: World Publishing Company, 1968.

Theobald, Robert. *Habit and Habitat.* Englewood Cliffs, N.J.: Prentice-Hall, 1972.

Thomas, Lewis, M.D. "Guessing and Knowing," *Saturday Review*, **55**, 52 (January 1973).

Thompson, William Irwin. "Planetary Vistas," *Harpers*, **243** (December 1971).

Tinbergen, Nikolaas. "Ethology and Stress Disease," *Science*, **185** (July 5, 1974).

Toffler, Alvin. *Future Shock.* New York: Random House, 1970.

Tolkien, J. R. R. *The Lord of the Rings.* Boston: Houghton Mifflin, 1965.

Tolstoy, Leo. "The Death of Ivan Illyich." In *Leo Tolstoi, Short Stories.* Margaret Wettlin, trans. Moscow: Progress Publishers, n.d.

Torrey, E. Fuller. "What Western Psychotherapists Can Learn from Witchdoctors," *American Journal of Orthopsychiatry*, **42,** 1 (January 1972). Reviewed in *Society*, **9,** 10 (September/October 1972).

Trussel, R. E.; Morehead, M. A.; et al. "A Study of the Quality of Hospital Care Secured by a Sample of Teamster Family Members in the New York Area." New York: Columbia University School of Public Health and Administration Medicine, 1972.

Tuma, May, and Tuma, N. "Schizophrenia—An Experimental Study of Five Treatment Methods," *British Journal of Psychiatry*, **111** (June 1965).

Udupa, K. N., and Singh, R. H. "The Scientific Basis of Yoga," *Journal of the American Medical Association*, **220,** 10 (June 5, 1972).

U.S. Department of Commerce, Bureau of the Census. "Projections of the

Population of the United States, by Age and Sex: 1970 to 2020," *Current Population Reports,* series P-25, no. 470. Washington, D.C.: U.S. Government Printing Office, 1971.

———. *Statistical Abstract of the United States, 1973.* 94th ed. Washington, D.C.: U.S. Government Printing Office, 1973.

U.S. Department of Health, Education, and Welfare. "Determinants of Expenditure for Physicians' Services in the U.S., 1948–68," DHEW Publication no. 73-3013, December 1972.

———. *National Institute of Alcohol Abuse and Alcoholism Report.* Washington, D.C.: U.S. Government Printing Office, February 1972.

———, National Institute of Health, National Cancer Institute. *National Cancer Program Plan.* Washington, D.C.: U.S. Government Printing Office, 1973.

———, Public Health Service. *Health Resources Statistics, 1972–73.* Washington, D.C.: U.S. Government Printing Office, 1973.

———, Public Health Service. *Mental Health.* Washington, D.C.: U.S. Government Printing Office, 1969.

———, Social Security Administration, Office of Research and Statistics. *Compendium of National Health Expenditures Data.* Washington, D.C.: U.S. Government Printing Office, 1972.

U.S. Department of Labor. *Work in America.* Washington, D.C.: U.S. Government Printing Office, 1972.

U.S. Surgeon General. *The Health Consequences of Smoking, A Public Health Service Review, 1967.* Washington, D.C.: Department of Health, Education, and Welfare, and Public Health Service, 1967.

U.S. Surgeon General. *Report on Smoking and Health.* Washington, D.C.: U.S. Government Printing Office, 1964.

Valentine, Thomas. *Psychic Surgery.* Chicago: Henry Regnery Company, 1975.

Virchow, Rudolf. *Cellular Pathology.* Frank Chance, trans. Ann Arbor, Mich.: Edwards Bros., 1940.

Vithoulkas, George. *Homeopathy: Medicine of the New Man.* New York: Avon, 1971.

Wallace, Robert K., and Benson, Herbert. "The Physiology of Meditation," *Scientific American,* **226** (February 1972).

Watson, Lyall. *Supernature.* Garden City, N.Y.: Doubleday Anchor Books, 1973.

Weil, Andrew. *The Natural Mind.* Boston: Houghton Mifflin, 1973.

Westlake, Aubrey T., M.D. *The Pattern of Health.* Berkeley: Shambala Publications Inc., 1973.

Wheeler, Harvey, and Carlson, R. J. "The Pursuit of Well-Being." A paper prepared for the Center for the Study of Democratic Institutions, Santa Barbara, Calif., February 1973.

White, John W. "Acupuncture: The World's Oldest System of Medicine," *Psychic,* July 1972.

White, Kerr. "Medical Care and Medical Cure," *Milbank Memorial Fund Quarterly,* **50** (October 1972).

White, Kerr, M.D. et al. "International Comparisons of Medical Care Utilization," *New England Journal of Medicine,* **272** (1967).

————. "Medical Care Research on Health Service Systems," *Journal of Medical Education,* **42** (August 1967).

Williams, Greer. "Quality vs. Quantity in American Medical Education," *Science,* **153** (August 26, 1966).

Williams, Roger J. "You Are Biochemically Unique," *Intellectual Digest,* April 1974.

Williamson, John, M.D. "Evaluating Quality of Patient Care," *Journal of the American Medical Association,* **218,** 4 (October 25, 1971).

Wilson, Colin. *The Occult.* New York: Vintage Books, 1973.

Yankelovich, Daniel. "The New Naturalism," *Saturday Review,* **55** (April, 1972).

Zola, Irving K. "Medicine as an Institution of Social Control." A paper presented at the Medical Sociology Conference of the British Sociological Conference, Westen-Super Mare, November 5–7, 1971.

Index

290 Index